Keto Diet for Seniors

A practical guide to the ketogenic diet full of tips for the needs of seniors, with a bonus of 38 recipes

Dana Roberts

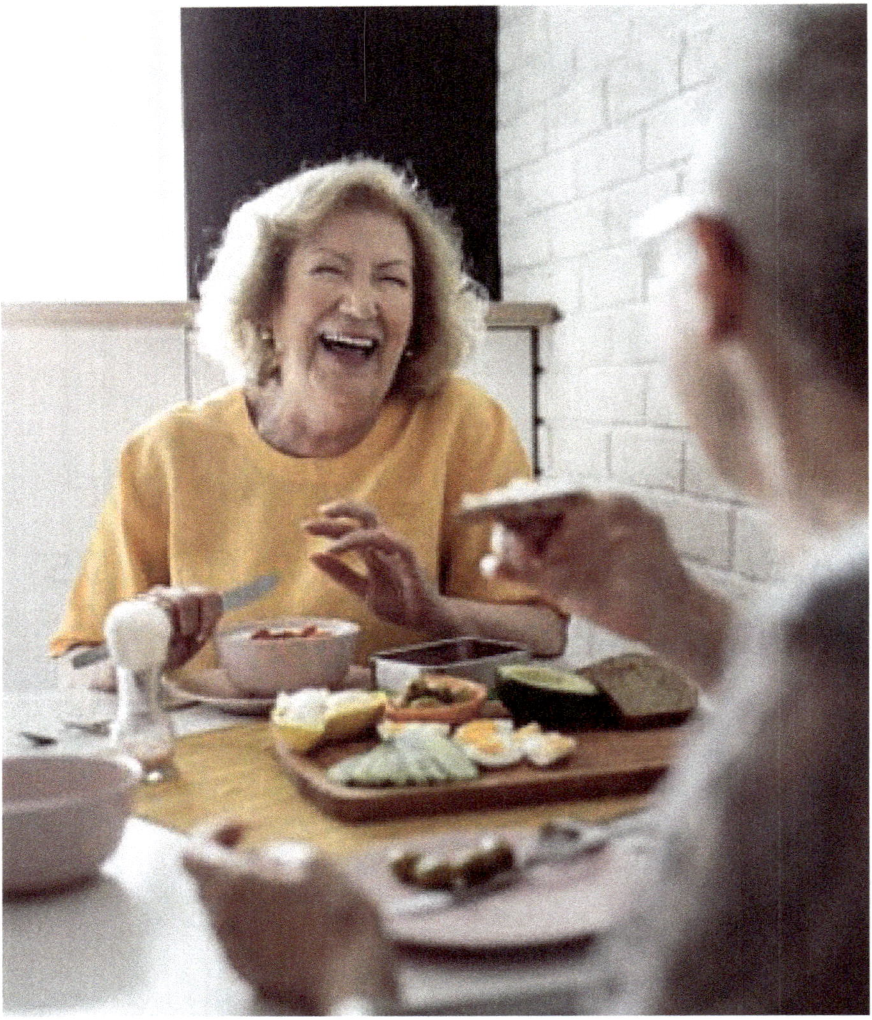

© Copyright 2020 by Dana Roberts - All rights reserved.

The following Book is reproduced below with the goal of providing information that is as accurate and reliable as possible. Regardless, purchasing this Book can be seen as consent to the fact that both the publisher and the author of this book are in no way experts on the topics discussed within and that any recommendations or suggestions that are made herein are for entertainment purposes only. Professionals should be consulted as needed prior to undertaking any of the action endorsed herein.

This declaration is deemed fair and valid by both the American Bar Association and the Committee of Publishers Association and is legally binding throughout the United States.

Furthermore, the transmission, duplication, or reproduction of any of the following work including specific information will be considered an illegal act irrespective of if it is done electronically or in print. This extends to creating a secondary or tertiary copy of the work or a recorded copy and is only allowed with the express written consent from the Publisher. All additional right reserved.

The information in the following pages is broadly considered a truthful and accurate account of facts and as such, any inattention, use, or misuse of the information in question by the reader will render any resulting actions solely under their purview. There are no scenarios in which the publisher or the original author of this work can be in any fashion deemed liable for any hardship or damages that may befall them after undertaking information described herein.

Additionally, the information in the following pages is intended only for informational purposes and should thus be thought of as universal. As befitting its nature, it is presented without assurance regarding its prolonged validity or interim quality. Trademarks that are mentioned are done without written consent and can in no way be considered an endorsement from the trademark holder.

Table of contents

Keto Diet for Women After 50

Body Changes after 50

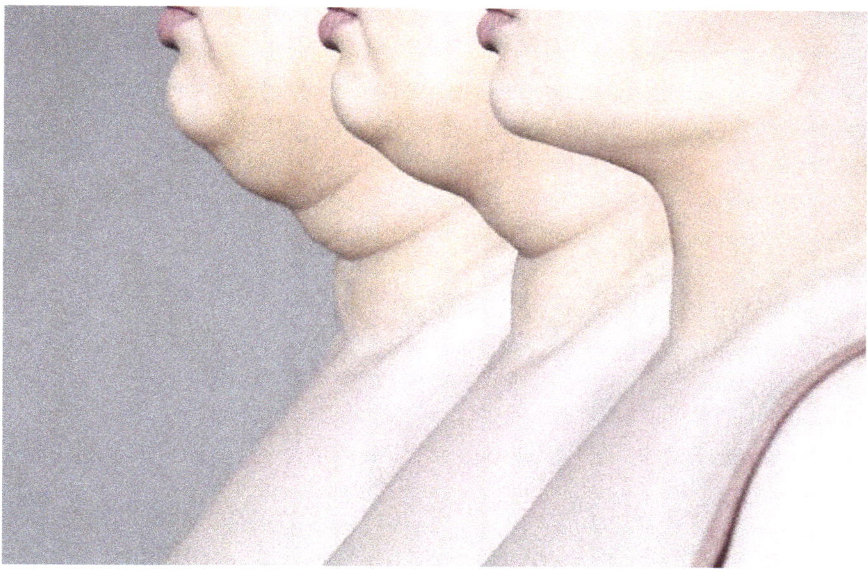

A living being keeps evolving throughout its life. Every age brings a new set of changes. Similarly, being over 50 always leads to significant changes in the body, which mainly includes:

1. **Lowering of the collagen production:** An important protein that helps in the rejuvenation of skin, hair, and nail cells. Thus, reduced collagen

production leads to wrinkled skin and poor hair growth.

2. **Dry skin:** When the skin loses its elasticity and collagen, it gets drier and rougher in appearance.
3. **The weakening of bones:** Another symptom of this age, as the bones no longer absorb calcium, and cartilage also suffers deterioration. It is particularly common among women, usually resulting in osteoporosis and arthritis.
4. **Menopause:** In women, menopause marks a significant change in the body. The reproductive system ceases to produce eggs, and the menstrual cycle stops for good. These changes occur under the influence of hormones and also lead to hormonal imbalances.
5. **Weight gain:** Reduced rate of metabolism at this age leads to obesity and weight gain. The calories are not actively consumed but rather stored in the body in one form or another to cause obesity.
6. **Enlarged heart:** High blood pressure and weakening of the muscle cells gradually leads to the enlargement of the heart. This may, in turn, cause more cardiac complications.
7. **Decreased memory recall:** The degeneration of brain cells is another effect of aging, and it leads to memory loss.

Benefits of the Keto Diet for People over 50

The above-discussed effects of aging can be reduced or controlled to some extent using the ketogenic diet. When the entire ketogenic lifestyle is followed along with dietary changes, it results in the following known benefits:

Accelerates Metabolism

As a person ages, it is the rate of metabolism that slows down with time. Metabolism is the sum total of all the processes that are carried out in the body. The building of new cells and elements, as well as the breaking of the existing agents into other elements. The fat-sourced high energy and release of ketones accelerate the rate of metabolism in the body.

Hormones Production

It is said that a woman's body is particularly more sensitive to dietary changes than the male body. It is because there are mainly several hormones that are at play in a woman's body. With a slight change in dietary habits and lifestyle, women can harness more benefits out of their fasting regime. Hormones in women's bodies are not only responsible for regulating the mood and internal body processes, but they also affect other systems in the body. The controlled release of energy and a healthy diet are responsible for maintaining the balance of estrogen and progesterone in the body.

PCOS

Polycystic ovarian syndrome is another common disorder that is prevalent among women of all ages, especially those over 50. PCOS cases are often the result of consistently high levels of insulin in the blood. Therefore, the ketogenic diet, due to its lowering of insulin effect, can treat or prevent PCOS to some extent. It can also control and counter the negative effects of PCOS in women.

Diabetes

Insulin resistance is a condition in which the body resists producing insulin. When the body fails to produce insulin, the pancreatic cells produce more insulin to lower the blood glucose levels. The excessive insulin production over a longer period of time ultimately wears out the pancreatic cells, and they lose the ability to produce necessary insulin levels, thus leading to diabetes. Since intermittent fasting can prevent insulin resistance by naturally lowering blood glucose levels, it also reduces the risks of diabetes. The ketogenic diet controls the insulin levels in the blood, thus prevents the risks of insulin resistance and diabetes.

Oxidative Stress

There are various chemical reactions that are occurring within the human body as a result of metabolism. These reactions produce millions of products and byproducts. Some chemical reactions produce free radicals, which are highly reactive in nature. When these radicals are left in the body for a longer duration of time, they can oxidize other elements in the cells and mingle with the natural cell cycle, ultimately leading to cell death. The cumulative effect of those free radicals is known as oxidative stress. When this stress increases, it can negatively affect human health. Ketones produced through ketosis work as antioxidants, which removes the free radicals and toxins from the body.

Cures Cancer

The ketogenic diet also improves the immune system, which helps patients to fight against all sorts of diseases, especially cancer. When the body undergoes ketosis, there is an increased production of lymphocytes that kills the pathogens, or agents, that may lead to cancer. Several cancer treatments also use this natural immune system to fight against the cancerous cells.

Inflammation

Inflammation is the swelling of body tissues and organs for any practical reason. In women over the age of 50, inflammation can result from hormonal or electrolyte imbalance. Accumulation of uric acid, high sugar, and cholesterol levels may also cause inflammation. Diseases like osteoporosis, or arthritis, which are common among women, also cause inflammation. Similarly, inflammation can also occur in the brain due to Alzheimer's or dementia. In any case, inflammation is always painful and health-damaging. Ketosis can help the body fight against the agents, causing inflammation. It promotes the immune system to increase its productivity. The damaged cells, which cause inflammation in the surrounding area, are then actively removed through autophagy to clean the body and repair it.

Weight Loss

Finally, weight loss is the most promising and obvious advantage of the ketogenic diet. Women over 50 years of age actively seek the keto diet to lose weight. It can reduce two to three pounds of weight within a week.

Ketogenic Diet and Menopause

Menopause always results in great stress for every woman, as there are several physical and psychological changes a woman goes through. The effects of menopause vary for each woman; it all depends on age, genetic makeup, living conditions, and diet. Menopause is characterized by the following known effects:

Insulin resistance

Poor Sleep

Weight gain

Brain fog

Dry skin and hair

Stress reactive

Hot flashes

Mood swings

Increased risk for heart disease

The weight gain alone can lead to further complications and severing of other symptoms like insulin resistance, lack of sleep, hot flashes, etc. During menopause, the fluctuation of the two hormones, estrogen, and progesterone, makes the body more stress reactive and insulin resistant. The disadvantage of being insulin resistant is that there will always be high blood glucose levels, which will lead to diabetes. All such effects of menopause can be prevented by switching to the ketogenic diet.

Common Mistakes and How to Fix Them

Every beginner is prone to commit some mistakes since the ketogenic diet is not a simple diet. It requires vigilant and careful meal planning and a great understanding of the diet. Here are common mistakes that people usually commit while following the ketogenic lifestyle.

Not Looking for the Hidden Carbs

Where people mostly look for and avoid the most obvious forms of carbs as sugars, grains, and beans, they fail to look out for hidden carbs that are largely present in processed food and market-packed products. Many food products that even say they are sugar-free may also contain a high amount of carbohydrates. By not avoiding such ingredients, people fail to achieve the results of ketosis. Therefore, practice the habit of reading the labels of all the food products and do not just rely on product tags.

Ignoring Nutritional Needs

Most women opt for a ketogenic diet only to lose weight. In this struggle of weight loss, they may turn a blind eye towards their nutritional needs. Controlling the carb intake does not mean depriving the body of what it needs to function properly. Therefore, meeting nutritional needs is imperative in this regard. Consume all the macro and micronutrients in your diet. Fibers, vitamins, minerals, and phytonutrients are as important as the proteins and fats for optimal brain and body function. The meal should contain a good amount of fats and protein to meet the needs of the body in the absence of carbohydrates.

Poor Hydration

When the body is in the state of ketosis, it loses water through increased urination. Dehydration can lead to electrolyte imbalance in the body. Therefore, it is very important to constantly hydrate yourself. The dieter must constantly drink water or other low-carb juices and smoothies to keep the body hydrated.

Avoiding Workouts

Most people over the age of 50 consider themselves too old to exercise as they feel weak in the bones and experience the lowering of metabolism. But exercise is proven crucial in harnessing the benefits of a ketogenic diet. A light and simple exercise routine are important to prepare the body for ketosis and the changes that come along with it.

No Monitoring of the Changes

Without keeping track of the changes that your body experiences after opting for the ketogenic diet, one can't really maintain this healthy routine. Most people complain that they have not experienced any change after the ketogenic diet, which is mainly because of the fact that they lose track of the new dietary routine they planned to follow. With constant monitoring, a person can also keep a check on his health conditions. Any signs of discomfort and negative effects should also be looked for.

Nutritional Needs and Food Addiction

Eating healthy tends to get more critical as we age because aging comes with a direct connection to various changes, which also include decreased life quality, nutrient deficiencies, and reduced strength.

Aging can be linked to various changes in our body, along with thinner skin, loss of muscles, and less acid in the stomach. Many of these changes can make us prone to deficiency of nutrients, while the remaining can affect our life quality and senses. When stomach acid level tends to low, it can directly affect nutrient absorption such as calcium, vitamin B12, magnesium, and iron. Another well-known challenge that comes along with aging is the reduced requirement for calories. Unfortunately, this results in a nutritional dilemma. The older people require only a certain amount of some of the nutrients while taking fewer calories.

Luckily, opting for various types of whole foods and supplements can help us meet all our nutritional needs as we age.

Need for Fewer Calories and More Nutrients

The daily calorie need of a person depends on various factors such as muscle mass, weight, height, activity level, and many others. Older adults need fewer amounts of calories for maintaining their body weight as they move and exercise less. They also carry less muscle. If you keep on taking in the same quantity of calories every day that you used to take in your younger days, you will end up gaining the extra amount of fat, specifically around the area of your belly. It is found mostly in postmenopausal women as they face a decline in estrogen levels, which promotes the storage of belly fat. However, even though older people require fewer calories, they also need high or even much higher levels of certain nutrients compared to younger individuals.

It makes it very essential for all older people to consume various natures of whole foods like fish, vegetables, and lean meats. All these healthy natures of staples can readily help in fighting with nutrient deficiencies without even affecting the waistline. Some of the nutrients that become essential as we age are vitamin D, vitamin B12, protein, and calcium.

Benefitting from More Protein

It is a common thing to lose strength and muscles as we age. An average adult loses about 4-8% of their total muscle mass every decade right after 30. This loss of power and muscle mass is known as sarcopenia. It is a vital cause of weakness, poor health, and fractures in older people. But, eating more amount of protein can help the body to regulate muscle and also fight sarcopenia. Eating more protein or even protein-based supplements can help slow down the loss of strength, increase total muscle mass, and contribute to building up more muscle.

More Fiber in the Diet

Constipation is the most common problem among most

aging and older people. It is more common in all those people who have crossed the mark of 65 years. The immediate solution for getting rid of constipation is to eat more fiber. Fiber can pass through our gut in an undigested form, helping the stool pass appropriately with the bowel's regular movements.

Need for More Vitamin D plus Calcium

These two are essential nutrients that are required for bone health. Calcium contributes to build up and maintain healthy bones with the help of Vitamin D. but, older people tend to absorb lesser amounts of calcium from their everyday diet.

Thus, with a deficiency of vitamin D and calcium, there will be a loss of bones with a high risk of having fractures. It is essential to consume all those food items rich in these nutrients. You can get calcium from various food items such as leafy vegetables and dairy products. Vitamin D can be found in multiple types of fish, such as herring and salmon. Older people can also consume vitamin D supplements, such as cod liver oil.

More Need of Vitamin B12

Older people are most likely to develop conditions that reduce stomach acid production, thus resulting in less absorption of vitamin B12 from food items. Atrophic gastritis is one of the states that can lead to this. For overcoming this, older people need to take supplements of vitamin B12, or they can also eat meals that are rich in vitamin B12.

Other Important Nutrients

Various other nutrients are required as you age. Let's have a look at them:

Potassium: Higher intake of potassium is often linked with reduced risk of high blood pressure, osteoporosis, kidney stones, and heart diseases. All of these disorders are very common among older people.

Omega-3 fatty acid: Heart disease is the prime cause of death among older people. It has been found that omega-3 fatty acid helps in lowering the risk factors of heart disease such as triglycerides and high blood pressure.

Iron: Iron deficiency is widespread in older people. In turn, it results in anemia, which is a condition in which there is not enough oxygen supplied to the body by the blood.

Magnesium: It is an essential mineral of the body. It helps in the digestion process, which tends to get disturbed with age.

These nutrients can be easily obtained by following a proper diet rich in vegetables, fruits, lean meat, and fish. The diet that you are going to choose will be affecting your lifestyle and health. A proper diet will also be affecting your mental health and functioning of the same. So, as you make up your diet, make sure that it contains all your required nutrients and the right propositions.

Tips for Seniors

Here are some tips to follow to achieve the desired goals:

Learn How to Count Your Macros

This is especially important at the start of your journey. As time goes by, you will learn how to estimate your meals without using a food scale.

Prepare Your Kitchen for Your Keto-friendly Foods

Once you've made a choice, it's time to get rid of all the foods in your kitchen that aren't allowed in the keto diet. To do this, check the nutritional labels of all the food items. Of course, there's no need to throw everything away. You can donate foods you don't need to food kitchens and other institutions that give food to the needy.

Purchase Some Keto Strips for Yourself

These are important so you can check your ketone levels and track your progress. You can purchase keto strips in pharmacies and online. For instance, some of the best keto strips available on Amazon are Perfect Keto Ketone Test

Strips, Smackfat Ketone Strips, and One Earth Ketone Strips.

Find an Activity You Enjoy

When you have done enough exercise, you will know what activities you like. One way to encourage yourself to exercise more regularly is by making it entertaining than a chore. If possible, stick to your favorite activities, and you can get the most out of your exercises. Keep in mind that the activities you enjoy may not be effective or needed, so you need to find other exercises to compensate for, which you may not enjoy. For instance, if you like jogging, you can work your leg muscles, but your arms are not involved. So, you need to do pushups or other strength training exercises.

Check with a Healthcare Provider

Your dietitian can tell you whether a keto diet would work. Still, it helps to check in with your healthcare provider to ensure that you do not have any medical condition that prevents you from losing weight, such as hypothyroidism and polycystic ovarian syndrome. It helps to know well in advance whether your body is even capable of losing fat in the first place before you commit and see no result, right?

Hydrate Properly

That means drinking enough water or herbal tea and ditch sweetened beverages or other drinks that contain sugar altogether. Making the transition will be difficult for the first few weeks, but your body will be thanking you for it. There is nothing healthier than good old plain water, and the recommended amount is 2 gallons a day.

Supplements

When you get older, your body starts to lose its ability to absorb certain nutrients, which leads to deficits. For example, vitamin B12 and folate are some of the most common nutrients that people over 50 lack. They have an impact on your mood, energy level, and weight loss rate.

Have the Right Mindset

Your mindset is one of the most important things you need to change when you've decided to follow the keto lifestyle. Without the right mindset, you might not stick with the diet long enough to enjoy all its benefits. Also, the proper mindset will keep you motivated to keep going no matter what challenges come your way.

Get Enough Sleep

Getting enough sleep helps your body regulate the hormones in your body, so try to aim for 7 to 9 hours of sleep a day. You can get more restful sleep by creating a nighttime routine that involves not looking at a computer, phone, or TV screen for at least 1 hour before bed. You can drink warm milk or water to help your body relax or even do 10 to 20 minutes of stretching to get a restful sleep.

Keep a Food Log

Then add the calories and divide by three to get an average. Now that you know how many takes, you can figure out how much you need to pay on average per day to reach your goals.

Lunch Recipes

Broccoli Muffins

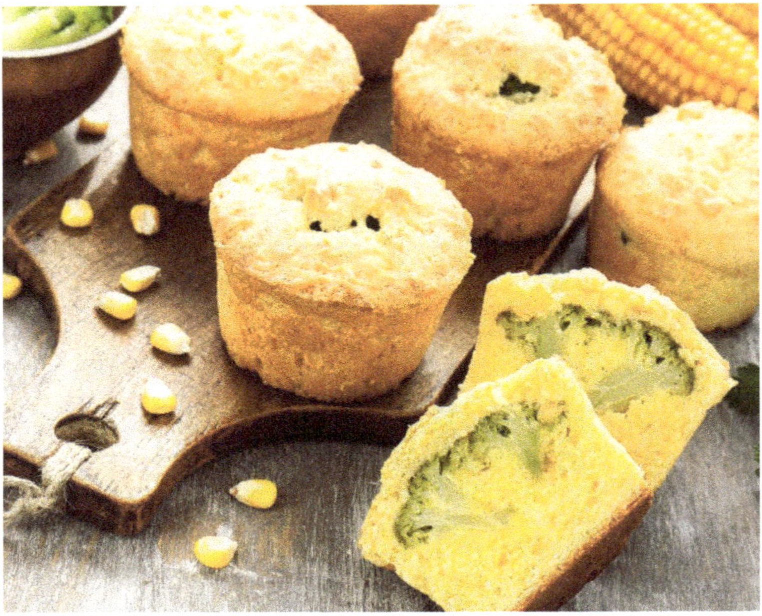

Preparation time: 15 Minutes

Cooking time: 20 Minutes

Servings: 5

Ingredients:

- 2 Tablespoons unsalted butter
- 6 Large organic eggs
- ½ Cup heavy whipping cream
- ½ Cup Parmesan cheese, grated
- Salt and ground black pepper, as required
- 1¼ Cups broccoli, chopped
- 2 Tablespoons fresh parsley, chopped
- ½ Cup Swiss cheese, grated

Directions:

1. Preheat your oven to 350°F.
2. Grease a 12-cup muffin tin.
3. In a bowl, add the eggs, cream, Parmesan cheese, salt, and black pepper, and beat until well combined.
4. Divide the broccoli and parsley in the bottom of each prepared muffin cup evenly. Top with the egg mixture, followed by the Swiss cheese.
5. Bake for about 20 minutes, rotating the pan once halfway through.
6. Remove from the oven and place onto a wire rack for about 5 minutes before serving.
7. Carefully invert the muffins onto a serving platter and serve warm.

Nutrition:

- Calories: 231 Net Carbs: 2g
- Total Carbs: 2.5g Fiber: 0.5g
- Sugar: 0.9g Protein: 13.5g

Eggs in Avocado Cups

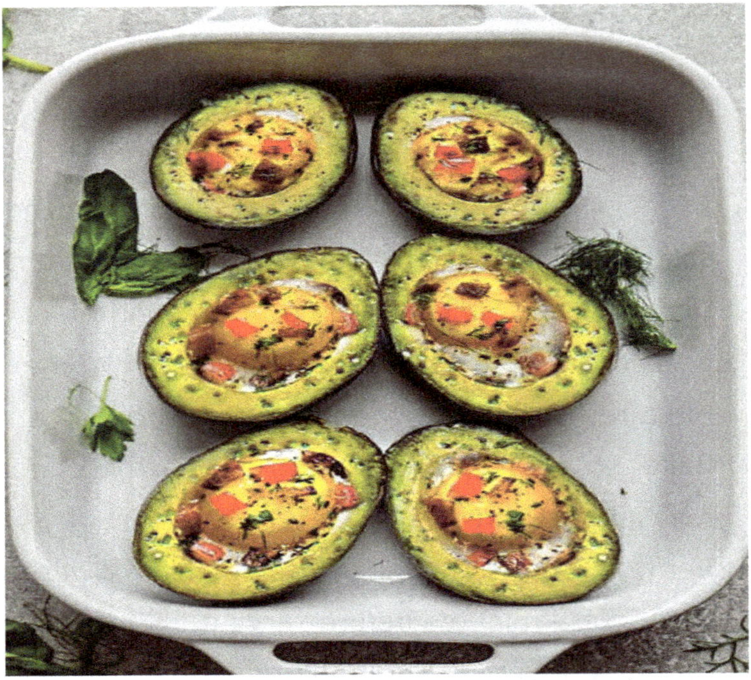

Preparation time: 10 Minutes

Cooking time: 20 Minutes

Servings: 4

Ingredients:

- 2 Ripe avocados, halved and pitted
- 4 Organic eggs
- Salt and ground black pepper, as required
- 4 Tablespoons cheddar cheese, shredded
- 2 Cooked bacon slices, chopped
- 1 Tablespoon scallion greens, chopped

Directions:

1. Preheat your oven to 400°F.
2. Carefully remove abut about two tablespoons of flesh from each avocado half. Place avocado halves into a small baking dish. Carefully crack an egg in each avocado half and sprinkle with salt and black pepper. Top each egg with cheddar cheese evenly.
3. Bake for about 20 minutes or until the desired doneness of the eggs.
4. Serve immediately with the garnishing of bacon and chives.

Nutrition:

- Calories: 343 Net Carbs: 2.2g
- Total Carbs: 7.9g Fiber: 5.7g
- Sugar: 0.8g Protein: 13.8g

Lemon Baked Salmon

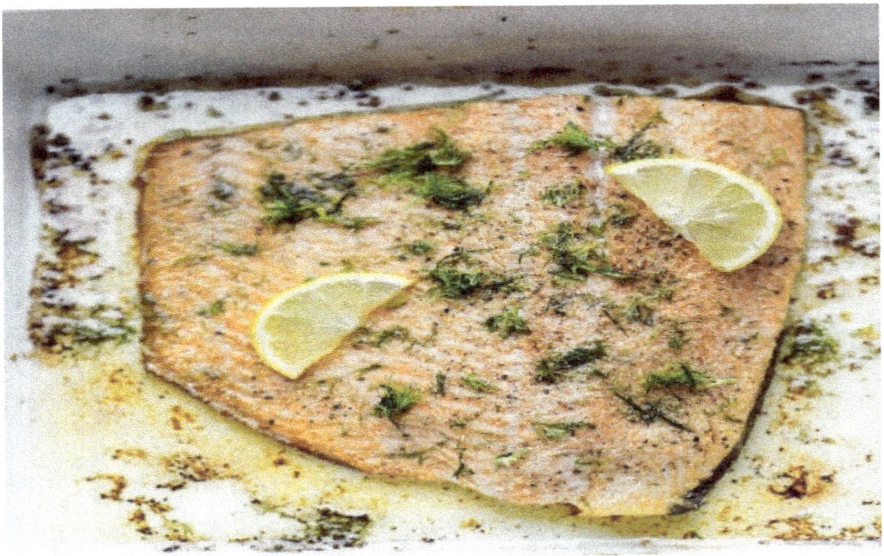

Preparation time: 10 Minutes

Cooking time: 30 Minutes

Servings: 4

Ingredients:

- 1 lb. Salmon
- 1 Tablespoon. olive oil
- Salt and pepper to taste
- 1 Tablespoon. butter
- 1 Lemon, thinly sliced
- 1 Tablespoon. lemon juice

Directions:

1. Preheat your oven to 400 degrees F.
2. Grease a baking dish with olive oil and place the salmon skin-side down.
3. Season the salmon with salt and pepper, then top with the lemon slices.
4. Slice half of the butter and place over the salmon.
5. Bake for 20 minutes or until the salmon flakes easily. Melt the remaining butter in a saucepan. When it starts to bubble, remove from heat and allow to cool before adding the lemon juice.
6. Drizzle the lemon butter over the salmon and servings warm.

Nutrition:

- Calories: 211kcal Carbs: 1.5g
- Fat: 13.5g Protein: 22.2g

Cauliflower Mash

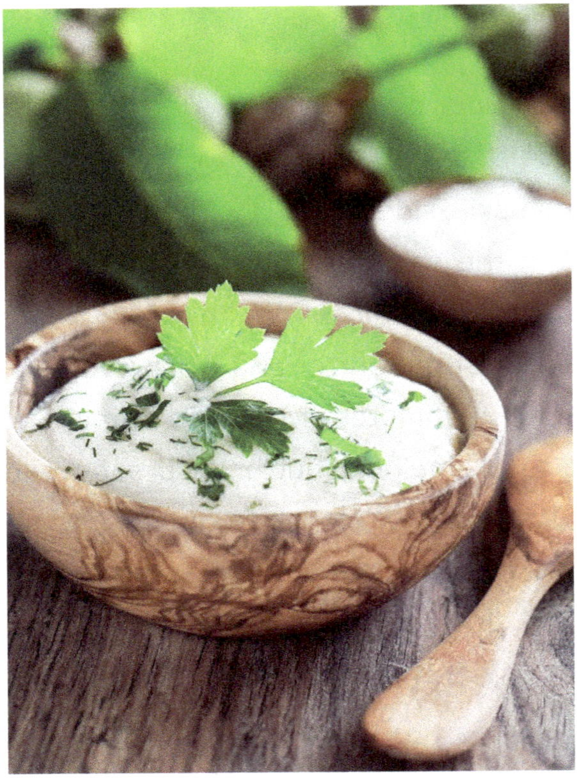

Preparation time: 10 Minutes

Cooking time: 5 Minutes

Servings: 8

Ingredients:

- 4 Cups cauliflower florets, chopped
- 1 Cup grated parmesan cheese
- 6 Tablespoons butter

- ½ Lemon, the juice and zest
- Salt and pepper to taste

Directions:

1. Boil the cauliflower in lightly salted water over high heat for 5 minutes or until the florets are tender but still firm.
2. Strain the cauliflower in a colander and add the cauliflower to a food processor.
3. Add the remaining ingredients and pulse the mixture to a smooth and creamy consistency.
4. Serve it with protein like salmon, chicken, or meatballs.
5. Can be refrigerated for up to 3 days.

Nutrition:

- Calories: 101kcal Carbs: 3.1g
- Fat: 9.5g Protein: 2.2g

Beef & Broccoli

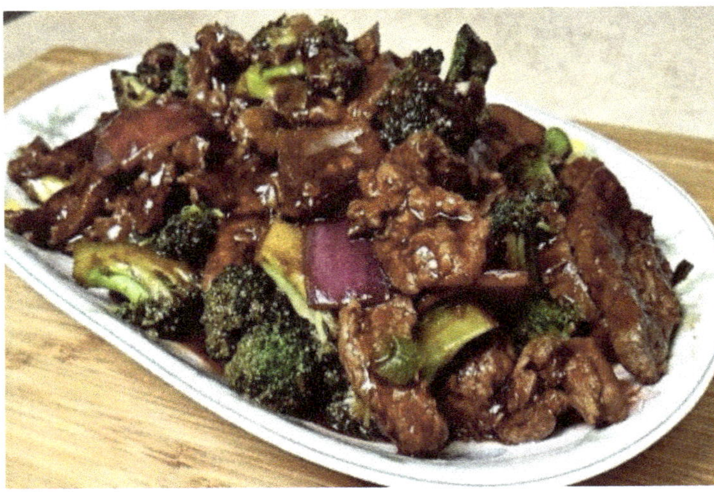

Preparation time: 10 Minutes

Cooking time: 15 Minutes

Servings: 2

Ingredients:

- ¼ Cup coconut amino, divided
- 1 Teaspoon garlic, minced and divided
- 1 Teaspoon fresh ginger, minced and divided
- 8oz. Beef, sliced thinly
- 1 ½ Tablespoon avocado oil, divided
- 2 ½ Cups broccoli, sliced into florets
- ¼ Cup beef stock, low sodium
- ½ Teaspoon sesame oil
- Salt to taste
- Sesame seeds

- Green onion, chopped

Directions:

1. In a bowl, mix the one tablespoon coconut amino with half of the ginger and garlic.
2. Marinate the beef into this mixture for 1 hour.
3. Cover with foil and place in the refrigerator.
4. Put one tablespoon oil in a pan over medium heat.
5. Add the broccoli and cook for 3 minutes.
6. Add the remaining ginger and garlic.
7. Cook for 1 minute.
8. Reduce heat.
9. Cover the pan with its lid.
10. Cook until the broccoli is tender but still a little crunchy.
11. Transfer the broccoli to a platter.
12. Increase the heat and add the remaining oil.
13. Add the beef and cook for 3 minutes.
14. Put the broccoli back.
15. In a bowl, mix the remaining coconut amino, broth, and sesame oil.
16. Pour into the pan.
17. Cook until the sauce has thickened.
18. Season with salt.
19. Garnish with sesame seeds and green onion.

Nutrition:

- Calories: 298
- Total Fat: 10g
- Saturated Fat: 3.1g
- Cholesterol: 101mg
- Sodium: 1989mg
- Total Carbohydrate: 12.2g
- Dietary Fiber: 4g
- Total Sugars: 2.7g
- Protein: 40g
- Potassium: 958mg

Cheddar Scramble

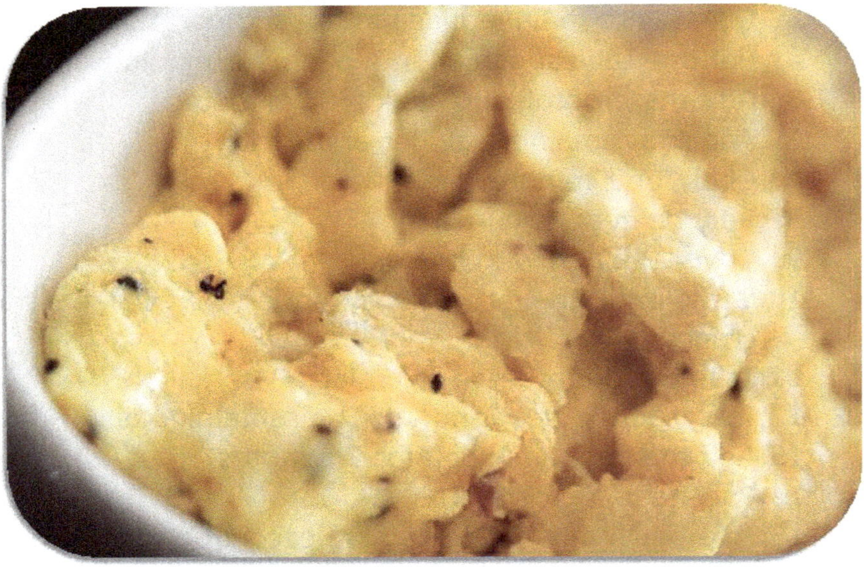

Preparation time: 10 Minutes

Cooking time: 8 Minutes

Servings: 2

Ingredients:

- 2 Tablespoons olive oil
- 1 Small yellow onion, chopped finely
- 12 Large organic eggs, beaten lightly
- Salt and ground black pepper, as required
- 4 Ounces cheddar cheese, shredded

Directions:

1. In a large wok, heat oil over medium heat and sauté the onion for about 4–5 minutes.
2. Add the eggs, salt, and black pepper and cook for about 3 minutes, stirring continuously.
3. Remove from the heat and immediately stir in the cheese.
4. Serve immediately.

Nutrition:

- Calories: 264
- Net Carbs: 1.8g
- Total Carbs: 2.1g
- Fiber: 0.3g
- Sugar: 1.4g
- Protein: 17.4g

Mustard-crusted Salmon

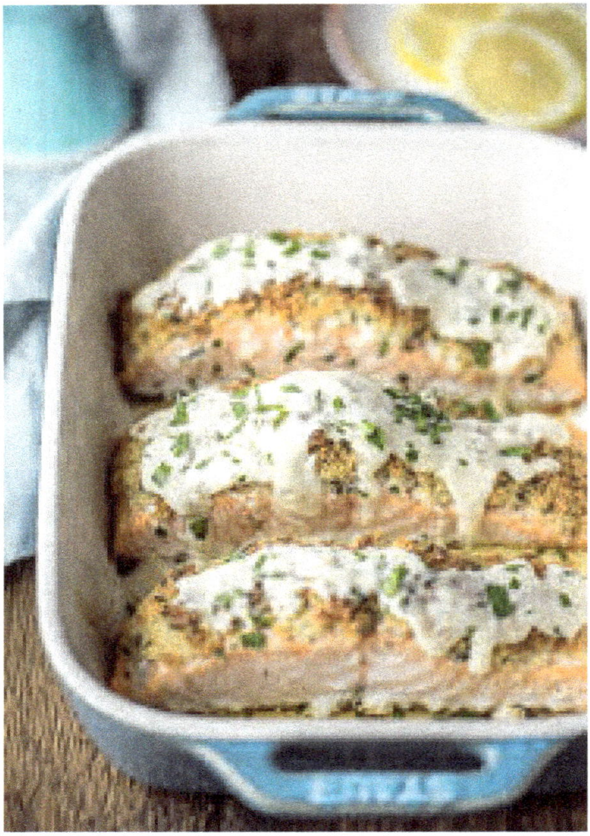

Preparation time: 15 Minutes

Cooking time: 15 Minutes

Servings: 4

Ingredients:

- 1 ¼ lb. Salmon fillets, cut into 4 portions
- 2 Tsp. lemon juice
- 2 Tbsp. stone-ground mustard
- Lemon wedges, for garnish

Directions:

1. In a large saucepan, put a trivet and pour a cup of water into the pan. Bring to a boil.
2. Place salmon in a heatproof dish that fits inside the saucepan and drizzle with olive oil. Season the salmon fillets with salt, pepper, and lemon juice. Sprinkle with mustard on top and garnish with lemon wedges on top—seal dish with foil.
3. Place the dish on the trivet inside the saucepan—cover and steam for 15 minutes.
4. Serve and enjoy.

Nutrition:

- Calories: 360 Fat: 24.8g
- Carbohydrates: 2.9g Protein: 29g

Halibut en Papillote

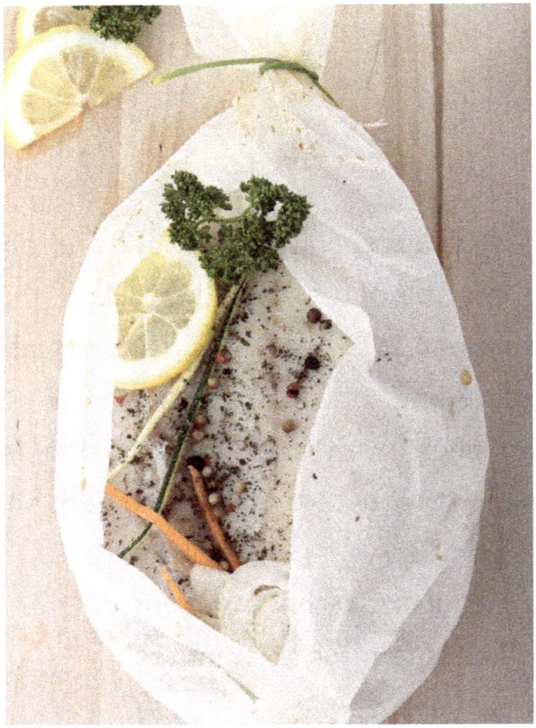

Preparation time: 10 Minutes

Cooking time: 15 Minutes

Servings: 4

Ingredients:

- 4 Halibut fillets
- ½ Tbsp. grated ginger
- 1 Cup chopped tomatoes
- 1 Shallot, thinly sliced
- 1 Lemon

Directions:

1. Slice lemon in half. Slice one lemon in circles.
2. In a small bowl, squeeze the other half of the lemon. Mix in grated ginger and season with pepper and salt.
3. Place a trivet in a large saucepan and pour a cup or two of water into the pan. Bring to a boil.
4. Get four large foil and place one fillet in the middle of each foil—season with fillet salt and pepper. Drizzle with olive oil. Add the grated ginger, tomatoes, and shallots equally. Fold the foil to generate a pouch and crimp the edges.
5. Place the foil containing the fish on the trivet—cover saucepan and steam for 15 minutes. Serve and enjoy in pouches.

Nutrition:

- Calories: 410 Fat: 32.3g
- Carbohydrates: 2.7g Protein: 20.3g

Keto Caesar Salad

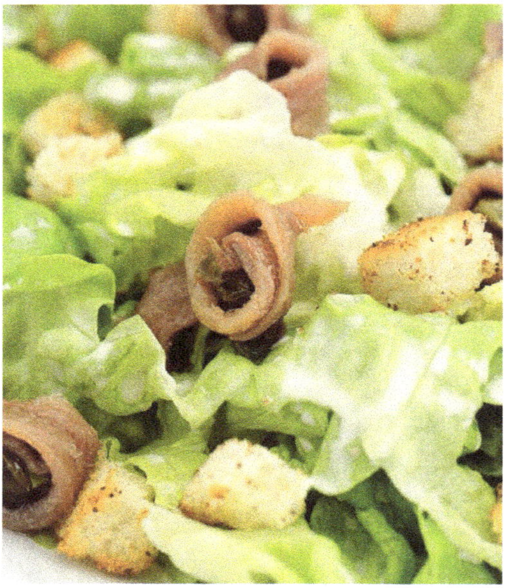

Preparation time: 15 Minutes

Cooking time: 0 Minutes

Servings: 4

Ingredients:

- 1.5 Cups Mayonnaise
- 3 Tablespoons Apple Cider Vinegar
- 1 Teaspoon Dijon Mustard
- 4 Anchovy Fillets
- 24 Romaine Heart Leaves

- 4oz. Pork Rinds
- Parmesan

Directions:

1. Process the mayo with ACV, mustard, and anchovies into a blender. Prepare romaine leaves and pour the dressing. Top with pork rinds and serve.

Nutrition:

- Calories: 993kcal Net Carbs: 4g
- Fiber: 3g Fat: 86g Protein: 47g

Kale Chips

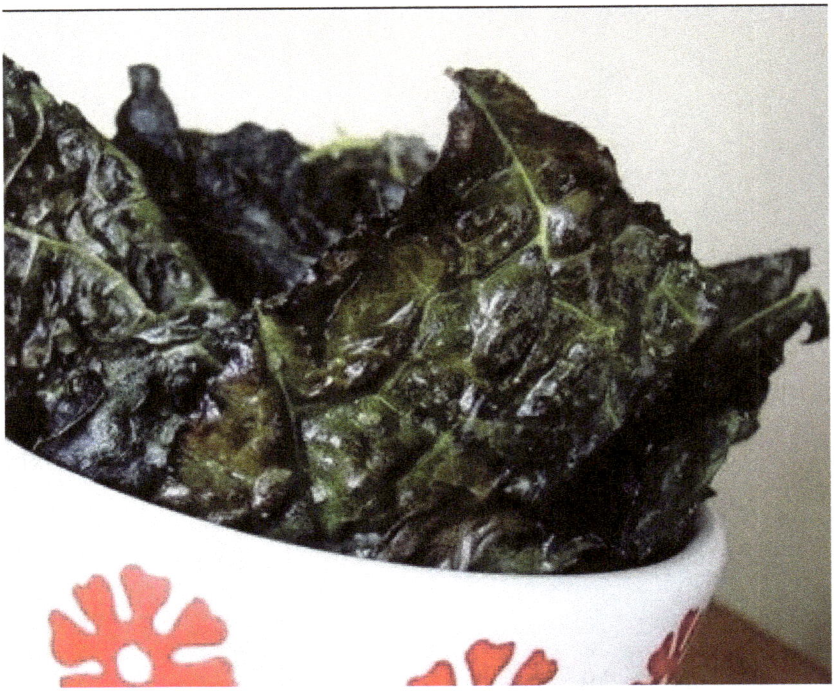

Preparation time: 5 Minutes

Cooking time: 12 Minutes

Servings: 2

Ingredients:

- 1 Bunch kale, removed from the stems
- 2 Tablespoons extra virgin olive oil
- 1 Tablespoon garlic salt

Directions:

1. Preheat your oven to 350 degrees F.
2. Coat the kale with olive oil.
3. Arrange on a baking sheet. Bake for 12 minutes. Sprinkle with garlic salt.

Nutrition:

- Calories: 100 Total Fat: 7g 9%
- Saturated Fat: 1g 5%
- Cholesterol: 0mg 0%
- Sodium: 30mg 1%
- Total Carbohydrate: 8.5g 3%
- Dietary Fiber: 1.2g 4%
- Total Sugars: 0.5g Protein: 2.4g
- Calcium: 92mg 7% Iron: 1mg 6%
- Potassium: 352mg

Bacon Mozzarella & Avocado

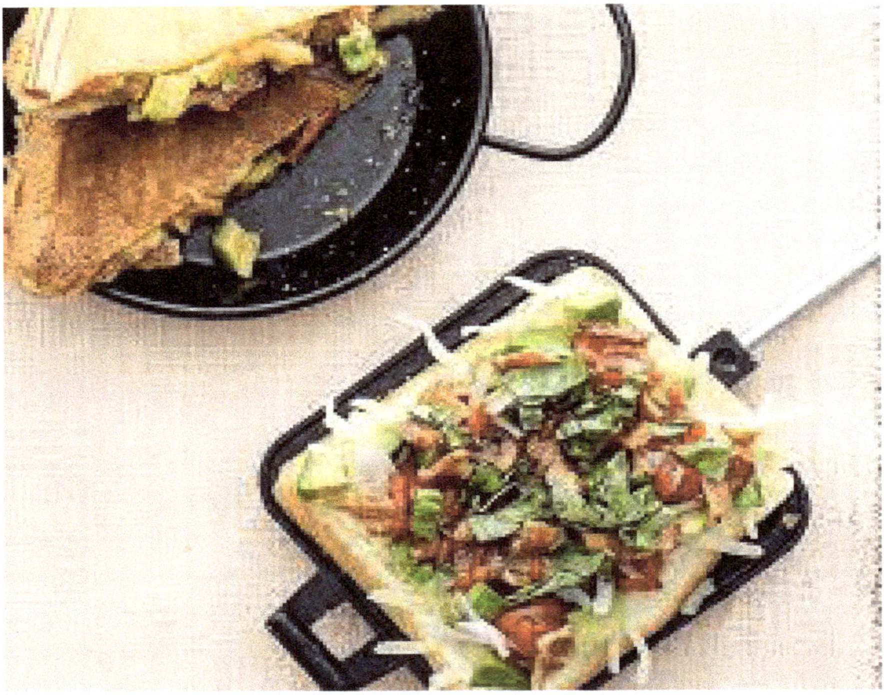

Preparation time: 15 Minutes

Cooking time: 15 Minutes

Servings: 2

Ingredients:

- 3 Slices bacon
- 1 Cup mozzarella cheese, shredded
- 6 Eggs, beaten
- 2 Tablespoons butter
- ½ Avocado

- 1oz. Cheddar cheese, shredded
- Salt and pepper to taste

Directions:

1. Fry the bacon in a pan until crispy.
2. Transfer to a plate and set aside.
3. Place the mozzarella cheese in the pan and cook until the edges have browned.
4. Cook the eggs in butter.
5. Stuff mozzarella with scrambled eggs, bacon, and mashed avocado.
6. Sprinkle cheese on top.
7. Season with salt and pepper.

Nutrition:

- Calories: 645 Total Fat: 53.6g
- Saturated Fat: 21.9g Cholesterol: 575mg
- Sodium: 1101mg
- Total Carbohydrate: 6.5g
- Dietary Fiber: 3.4g Total Sugars: 1.4g
- Protein: 35.8g Potassium: 600mg

Keto Buffalo Chicken Empanadas

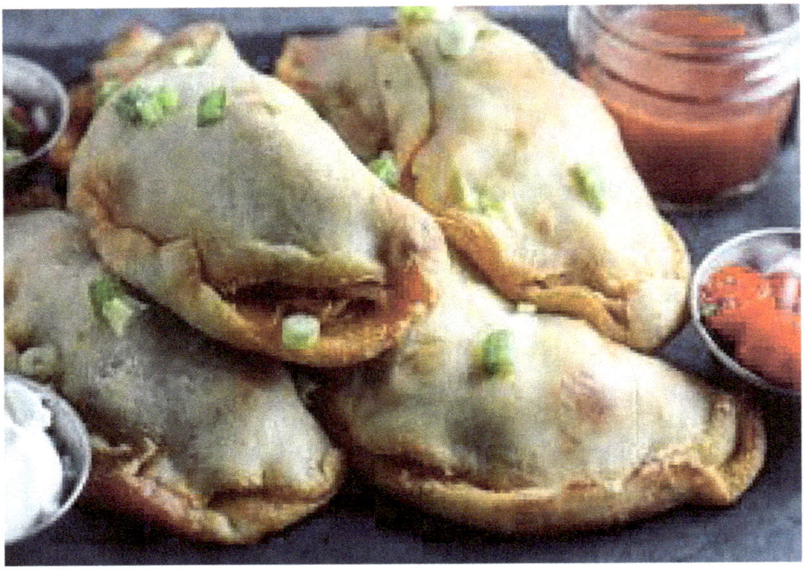

Preparation time: 20 Minutes

Cooking time: 30 Minutes

Servings: 6

Ingredients:

For the empanada dough:

- 1 ½ Cups mozzarella cheese
- 3oz. Cream cheese
- 1 Whisked egg
- 2 Cups almond flour

For the buffalo chicken filling:

- 2 Cups shredded chicken

- 2 Tablespoons Butter
- 0.33 Cup Hot Sauce

Directions:

1. Warm-up oven, 425-degrees.
2. Microwave the cheese & cream cheese within 1-minute. Stir the flour and egg into the dish.With another bowl, combine the chicken with sauce and set aside.
3. Cover a flat surface with plastic wrap and sprinkle with almond flour.
4. Grease a rolling pin, press the dough flat.
5. Make the circle shapes out of this dough with a lid. Portion out a spoonful of filling into these dough circles. Fold the other half over to close up into half-moon shapes. Bake within 9 minutes. Serve.

Nutrition:

- Net carbs: 20g Fiber: 0g
- Fat: 96g Protein: 74g Calories: 1217kcal

Pepperoni and Cheddar Stromboli

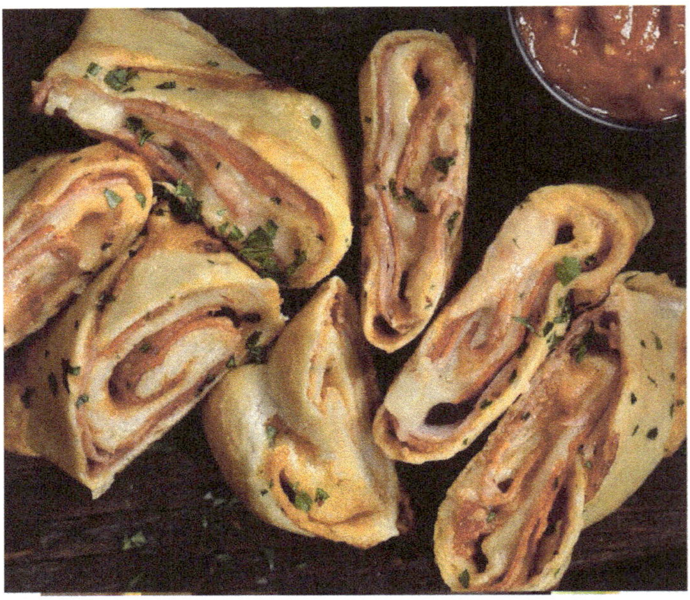

Preparation time: 15 Minutes

Cooking time: 20 Minutes

Servings: 3

Ingredients:

- Cups Mozzarella Cheese
- 0.25 Cup Almond Flour
- 3 Tablespoons Coconut Flour
- 1 Teaspoon Italian Seasoning
- 1 Egg - 6oz. Deli Ham

- 2oz. Pepperoni
- 4oz. Cheddar Cheese
- 1 Tbsp. Butter
- 6 Cups Salad Greens

Directions:

1. Warm-up the oven, 400 degrees.
2. Melt the mozzarella—mix flours & Italian seasoning in a separate bowl.
3. Dump in the melty cheese and mix with pepper and salt.
4. Stir in the egg and process the dough. Pour it onto that prepared baking tray.
5. Roll out the dough. Cut slits that mark out four equal rectangles. Put the ham and cheese, then brush with butter and close up. Bake within 17 minutes. Slice and serve.

Nutrition:

- Net carbs: 20g Fiber: 0g Fat: 13g
- Protein: 11g Calories: 240kcal

Five-Spice Steamed Tilapia

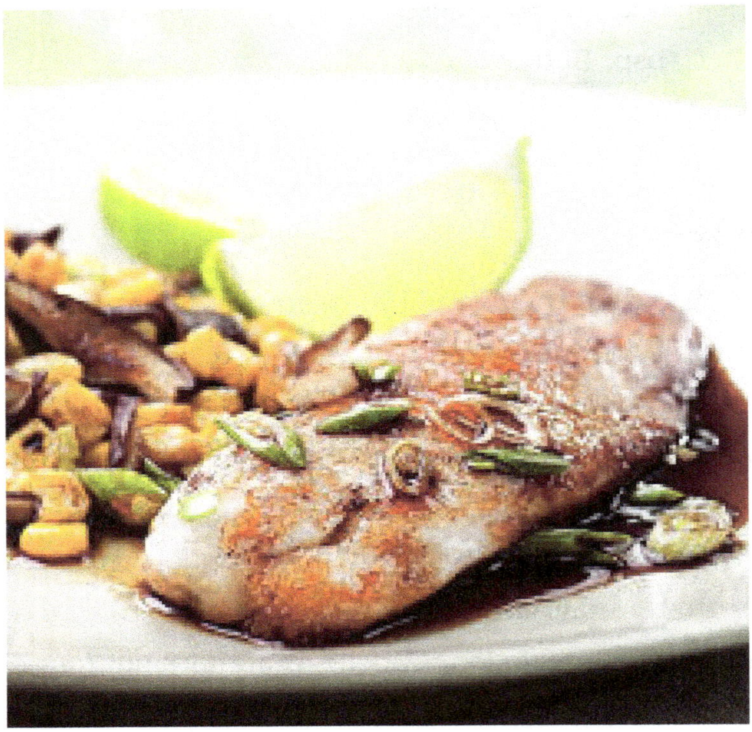

Preparation time: 15 Minutes

Cooking time: 15 Minutes

Servings: 4

Ingredients:

- 1lb. Tilapia fillets,
- 1 Tsp. Chinese five-spice powder
- 3 Tablespoons coconut oil
- 3 Scallions, sliced thinly

Directions:

1. In a large saucepan, place a trivet and pour a cup of water into the pan. Bring to a boil.
2. Place tilapia in a heatproof dish that fits inside a saucepan. Drizzle oil on tilapia. Season with salt, pepper, and Chinese five-spice powder. Garnish with scallions.
3. Seal dish with foil. Place the dish on the trivet inside the saucepan—cover and steam for 15 minutes.
4. Serve and enjoy.

Nutrition:

- Calories: 201 Fat: 12.3g
- Carbohydrates: 0.9g Protein: 24g

Shrimp and Cauliflower Jambalaya

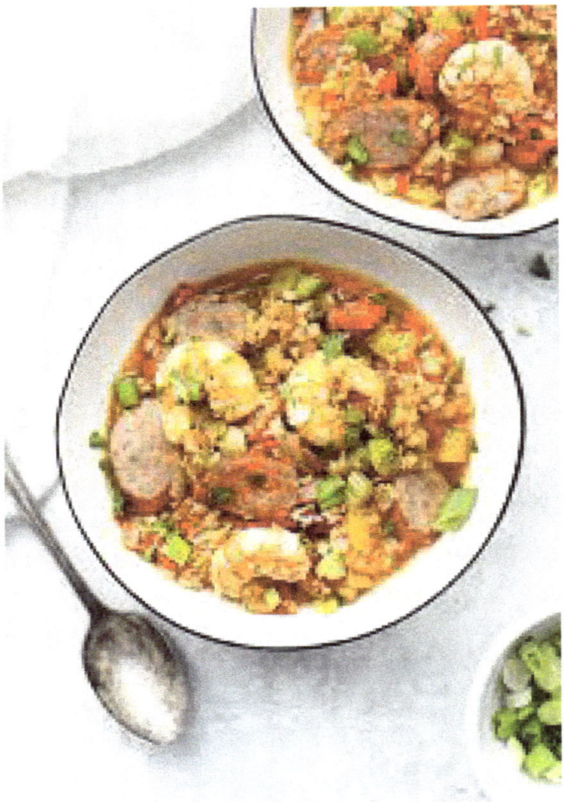

Preparation time: 20 Minutes

Cooking time: 15 Minutes

Servings: 4

Ingredients:

- 2 Cloves garlic, peeled and minced
- 1 Head cauliflower, grated

- 1 Cup chopped tomatoes
- 8oz. Raw shrimp, peeled and deveined
- 1 Tbsp. Cajun seasoning

Directions:

1. On medium-high fire, heat a non-stick saucepan for 2 minutes. To a pan, add oil and swirl to coat the bottom and sides. Heat oil for a minute.
2. Add garlic and sauté for a minute. Stir in tomatoes and stir fry for 5 minutes. Add water and deglaze the pan.
3. Add remaining ingredients. Season generously with pepper.
4. Increase fire to high and stir fry for 3 minutes.
5. Lower the fire, cover, and cook for 5 minutes.
6. Serve and enjoy.

Nutrition:

- Calories: 314 Fat: 22.25g
- Carbohydrates: 7.8g Protein: 21.4g

Stuffed Chicken

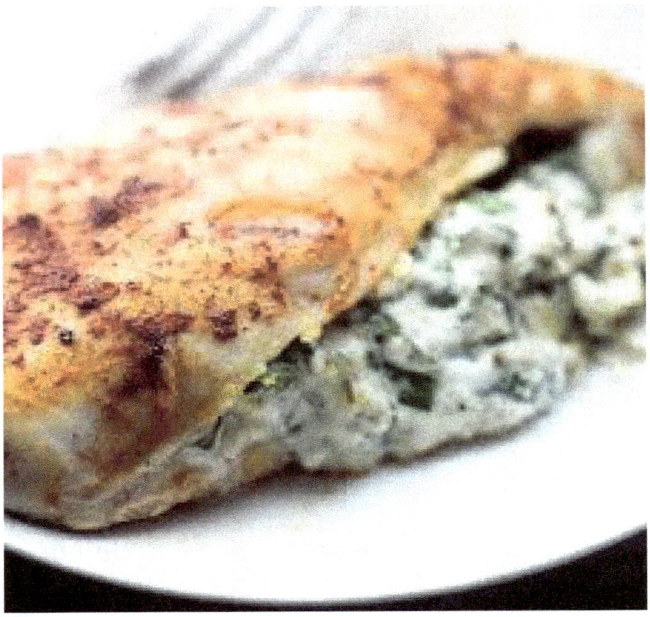

Preparation time: 10 Minutes

Cooking time: 25 Minutes

Servings: 2

Ingredients:

- 4 Chicken breasts, boneless, skinless butterfly cut
- ½ Cup frozen spinach
- 1/3 Cup feta cheese, crumbled
- 1/4 Teaspoon of black pepper and salt
- 2 Tablespoons of coconut oil
- 1 Cup Water

Directions:

1. Pound the chicken breast pieces into 1/4 inch thickness.
2. Butterfly cut the chicken pieces and set aside for further use.
3. Take a medium bowl and mix spinach, feta cheese, pepper, and salt.
4. Divide this mixture evenly by spooning it into the chicken breasts.
5. Close the chicken breast and secure with a toothpick.
6. Now, turn on the sauté mode of the instant pot and then add coconut oil to it.
7. Sear the chicken breast in batches until golden brown.
8. Then press the cancel button of the pot.
9. Set aside the chicken and go for the next steps.
10. Now pour the water into the same pot and scrape the bottom to remove the seasoning.
11. Now adjust the steamer rack in the pot and place chicken on top of the rack.
12. Adjust the timer to 15 minutes at high pressure.
13. Once the timer goes off, naturally release the steam. Serve the dish hot.

Nutrition:

- Calories: 742
- Total Fat: 40.6g
- Saturated Fat: 21.5g
- Iron: 4mg
- Potassium: 775mg

Curried Chicken with Instant Lemon

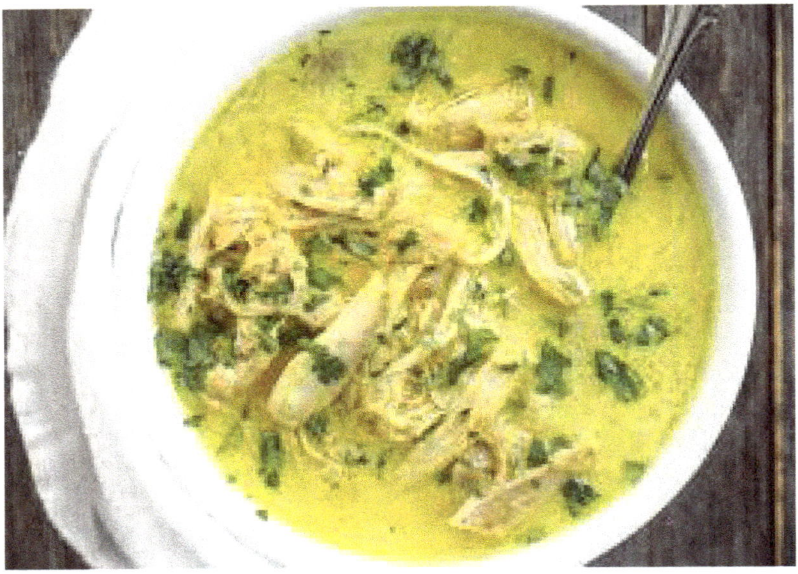

Preparation time: 10 Minutes

Cooking time: 25 Minutes

Servings: 6

Ingredients:

- 1 can Coconut Milk, full fat
- 1/4 cup Lemon juice - 1 Tsp. turmeric
- 6 Pcs. Chicken breasts or thighs
- 1 Tbsp. Curry Spice

Directions:

1. Set your instant pot on high heat.
2. Add all ingredients and set on the manual setting. Secure the vent sealing and cover. Set the timer for about 4 hours. Serve hot!

Nutrition:

- Calories: 321Kcal Fat: 15g
- Carbs: 1g Protein: 20g

Dinner Recipes

Seafood Casserole

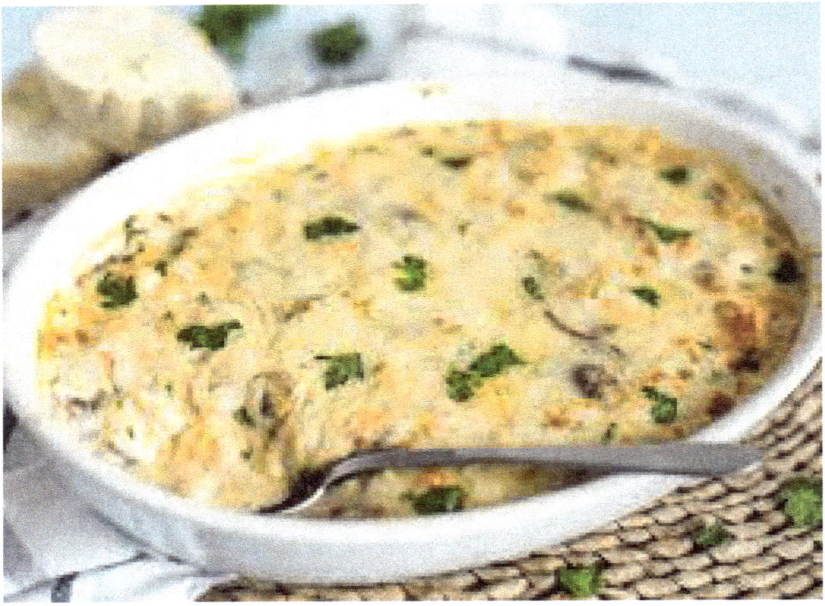

Preparation time: 20 Minutes

Cooking time: 36 Minutes

Servings: 6

Ingredients:

- 2 Cups of eggplant
- Bits of butter. Sliced and cut in1-inch
- 1 Tablespoon of olive oil
- 1/2 Small sweet onion
- 1 Tablespoon of minced garlic
- 1 Celery stalk
- 1/2 Red bell pepper
- 3 Tablespoons of freshly squeezed lemon juice
- 1 Tablespoon of hot sauce
- 1/4 Tablespoon of Creole Seasoning Mix (here)
- 1/2 Cup of white rice

- 1 Large egg
- 3 Ounces of cooked shrimp

Directions:

1. Cook the eggplant for 6 minutes in a small saucepan filled with water over medium-high heat.
2. Drain in a large bowl and set aside.
3. Grease and set aside an 8-by-13-inch butter baking dish. Heat the olive oil in a large pot over medium heat.
4. Drizzle the onion, garlic, celery, and pepper bell for about 3 minutes or until tender. In addition to the lemon juice, hot sauce, Creole seasoning, rice, and egg, add the sauteéd vegetables to the eggplant.
5. Remove to combine. Fold in the meat of the crab and shrimp.
6. In the casserole dish, spoon the casserole mixture and pat down the top. Bake for 26 to 40 minutes until the casserole is heated through and the rice is tender. Serve hot.

Nutrition:

- Fat: 3g
- Carbohydrates: 8g
- Phosphorus: 102 mg
- Potassium: 188mg
- Sodium: 236mg
- Protein: 12g

Herb Pesto Tuna

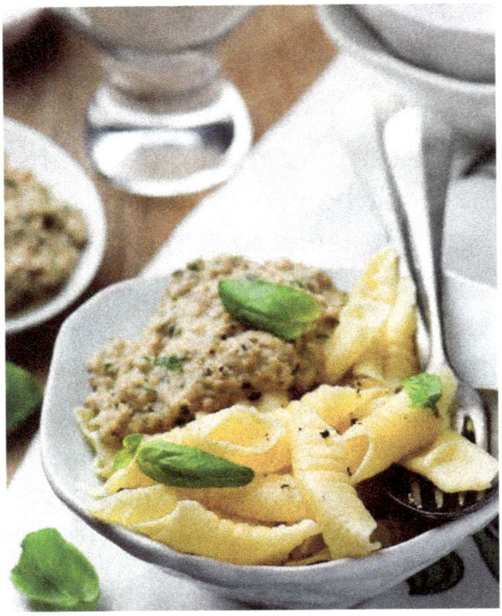

Preparation time: 10 Minutes

Cooking time: 10 Minutes

Servings: 3

Ingredients:

- 3 (3-ounce) Yellowfin tuna fillets
- 1 Tablespoon olive oil
- Freshly ground black pepper
- 1/4 Cup Herb Pesto (see here)
- 1 Lemon, cut into 8 thin slices

Directions:

1. Heat to medium-high barbecue. Add the olive oil to the fish and season each fillet with pepper. Cook it for 3 minutes.
2. Turn over the fish and top each piece using the herb slices. Grill until the tuna is cooked to medium-well for 6 to 6 minutes longer.

Modification of dialysis: The pesto adds to this recipe about 16mg of potassium. The tuna is the reason why the potassium recipe is high. Try this recipe with other fish like haddock or cod, but instead of putting it on the barbecue, broil the fish.

Nutrition:

- Fat: 2g
- Phosphorus: 236mg
- Sodium: 38mg

Grilled Calamari with Lemon and Herbs

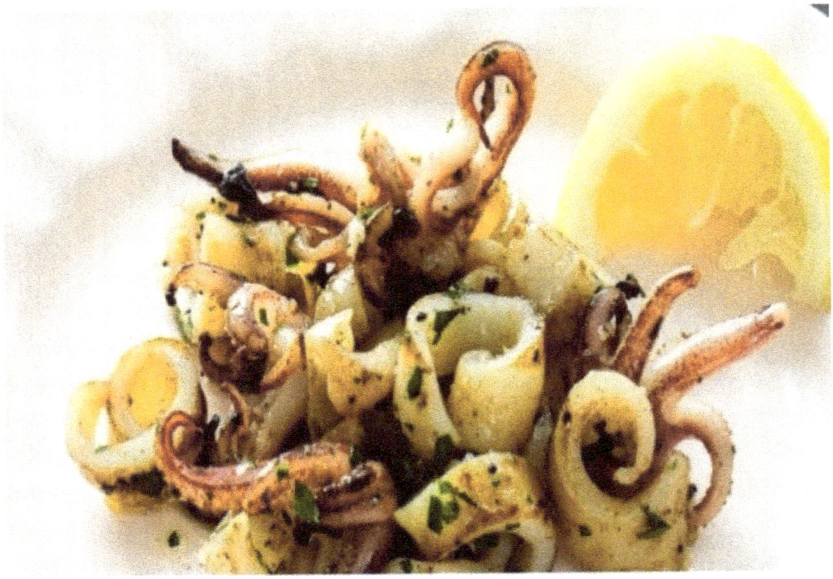

Preparation time: 10 Minutes

Cooking time: 3 Minutes

Servings: 3

Ingredients:

- 2 Tablespoons of olive oil
- 2 Tablespoons of freshly squeezed lemon juice
- 1 Tablespoon of chopped fresh parsley
- 1 Tablespoon of chopped fresh oregano
- 2 Tablespoons of minced garlic
- Pinch sea salt
- Pinch freshly ground black pepper
- 1/2 pound of cleaned calamari
- Lemon wedges, to be garnished

Directions:

1. In a large bowl, combine olive oil, lemon juice, petroleum, oregano, garlic, salt, and pepper.
2. In the bowl, add the calamari and stir to coat. Cover the bowl and cool the calamari to marinate for 1 hour.
3. Preheat the barbecue to medium-high. Grill the calamari for about 3 minutes, turning once, until firm and opaque. Serve with wedges of lemon.

Nutrition:

- Fat: 8g
- Carbohydrates: 2g
- Phosphorus: 128mg
- Potassium: 160mg
- Sodium: 68mg
- Protein: 3g

Traditional Chicken-Vegetable Soup

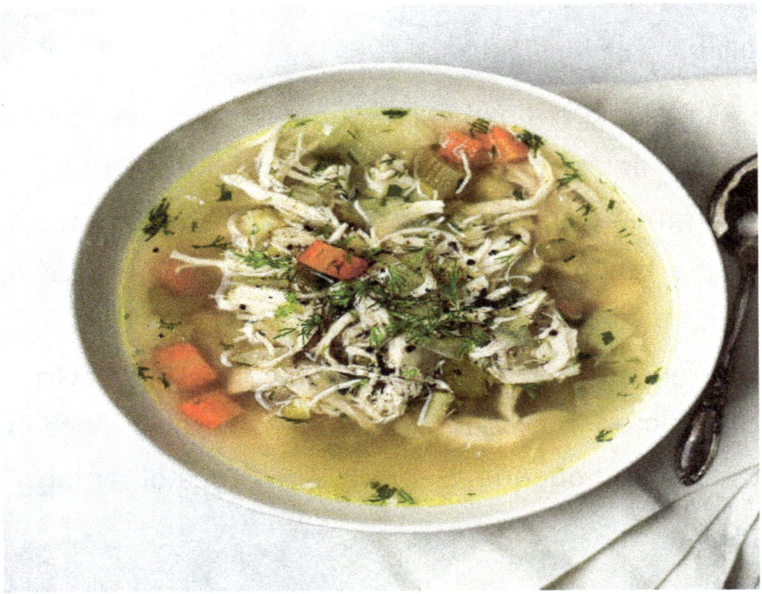

Preparation time: 20 Minutes

Cooking time: 36 Minutes

Servings: 2

Ingredients:

- 1 Tablespoon of unsalted butter
- 1/2 Sweet onion
- 2 Tablespoons of chopped garlic
- 2 Celery stalks
- 1 Carrot chopped
- 2 Cups of chicken breast chopped

- 1 Cup of Easy Chicken Stock
- 3 Cups of water
- 1 Tablespoon of freshly chopped thyme
- Black pepper freshly ground
- 2 Tablespoons of chopped fresh parsley

Directions:

1. Melt the butter in a large pot over medium heat. Sauté the onion and garlic for about 3 minutes until softened.
2. Add celery, carrot, chicken, stuffed chicken, and water. Bring the soup to a boil, reduce heat, and simmer until the vegetables are tender for about 40 minutes.
3. Add the thyme and cook the soup for 2 minutes. Season with pepper and serve with parsley on top.

Nutrition:

- Fat: 6g
- Carbohydrates: 2g
- Phosphorus: 108mg
- Potassium: 188mg
- Sodium: 62mg
- Protein: 16g

Shrimp Scampi with Garlic

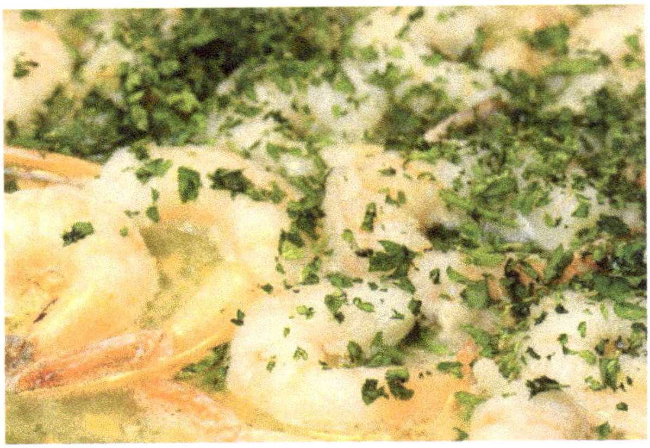

Preparation time: 5 Minutes

Cooking time: 10 Minutes

Servings: 4

Ingredients:

- 1 Pound shrimp
- 3 Tbsp. olive oil
- 1 Bulb shallot, sliced
- 4 Cloves garlic, minced
- ½ Cup Pinot Grigio
- 4 Tbsp. salted butter
- 1 Tbsp. lemon juice
- ½ Tsp. sea salt
- ¼ Tsp. black pepper

- ¼ Tsp. red pepper flakes
- ¼ Cup parsley, chopped

Directions:

1. Pour the olive oil into the heated frying pan. Add the garlic and shallots and fry for about 2 minutes.
2. Combine the Pinot Grigio, salted butter, and lemon juice. Pour this mix into the pan and cook for 5 minutes.
3. Put the parsley, black pepper, red pepper flakes, and sea salt into the pan and whisk well. Add the shrimp and fry until they are pink (about 3 minutes).

Nutrition:

- Calories: 344 Fat: 7g
- Carbohydrates: 7g Protein: 32g

Chinese Pork Bowl

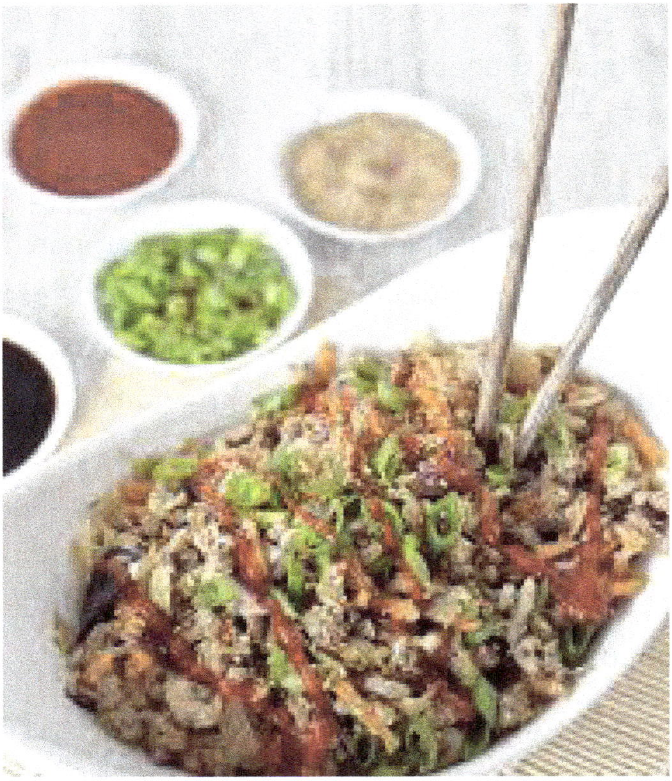

Preparation time: 5 Minutes

Cooking time: 15 Minutes

Servings: 4

Ingredients:

- 1¼ Pounds pork belly, cut into bite-size pieces
- 2 Tbsp. tamari soy sauce
- 1 Tbsp. rice vinegar

- 2 Cloves garlic, smashed
- 3oz. Butter
- 1 Pound Brussels sprouts, rinsed, trimmed, halved, or quartered
- ½ Leek, chopped
- Salt and ground black pepper, to taste

Directions:

1. Fry the pork over medium-high heat until it is starting to turn golden brown.
2. Combine the garlic cloves, butter, and Brussels sprouts. Add to the pan, whisk well and cook until the sprouts turn golden brown.
3. Stir the soy sauce and rice vinegar together and pour the sauce into the pan.
4. Sprinkle with salt and pepper.
5. Top with chopped leek.

Nutrition:

- Calories: 993 Fat: 97g
- Carbs: 7g Protein: 19g

Slow Roasting Pork Shoulder

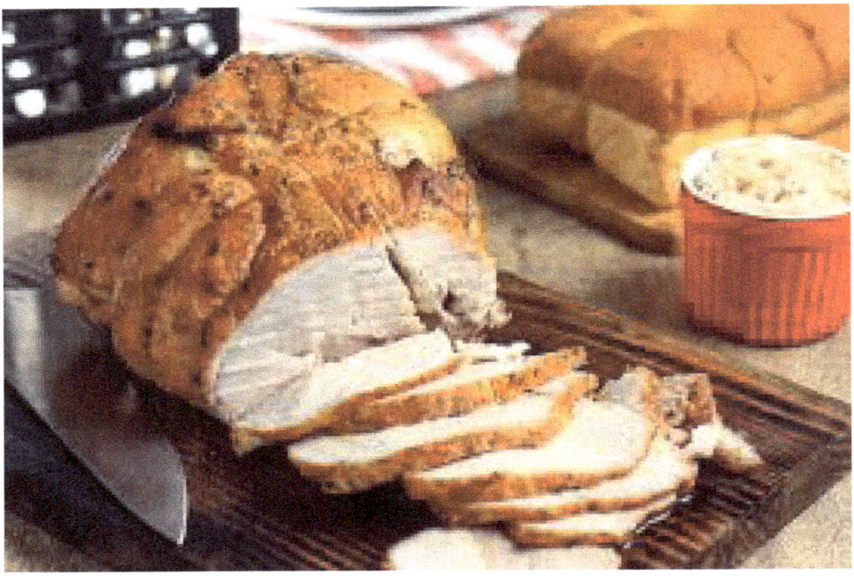

Preparation time: 15 Minutes

Cooking time: 7 Hours

Servings: 8

Ingredients:

- 3 lb. Pork shoulder
- 8 Garlic cloves, minced
- ½ C. fresh lemon juice
- 2 Tbsp. olive oil
- 1 Tbsp. low-sodium soy sauce
- 1/3 C. homemade chicken broth

Directions:

1. In a nonreactive baking dish, arrange the pork shoulder, fat side up.
2. With the tip of a knife, score the fat in a crosshatch pattern.

3. In a bowl, add the garlic, lemon juice, soy sauce, and oil and mix well.
4. Place the marinade over pork and coat well.
5. Refrigerate for about 4-6 hours, flipping occasionally.
6. Preheat the oven to 3150 F. Lightly grease a large roasting pan.
7. With paper towels, wipe marinade off the pork shoulder.
8. Arrange the pork shoulder into a prepared roasting pan, fat side up.
9. Roast for about 3 hours.
10. Remove from the oven and pour the broth over the pork shoulder.
11. Roast for about 3-4 hours, basting with pan juices, after every 1 hour.
12. Remove from the oven and place the pork shoulder onto a cutting board for about 30 minutes.
13. With a sharp knife, cut the pork shoulder into the desired size slices and serve.

Nutrition:

- Calories per serving: 537
- Carbohydrates: 1.5g
- Protein: 40.2g
- Fat: 40.1g
- Sugar: 0.5g
- Sodium: 261mg
- Fiber: 0.1g

Skillet Cabbage Tacos

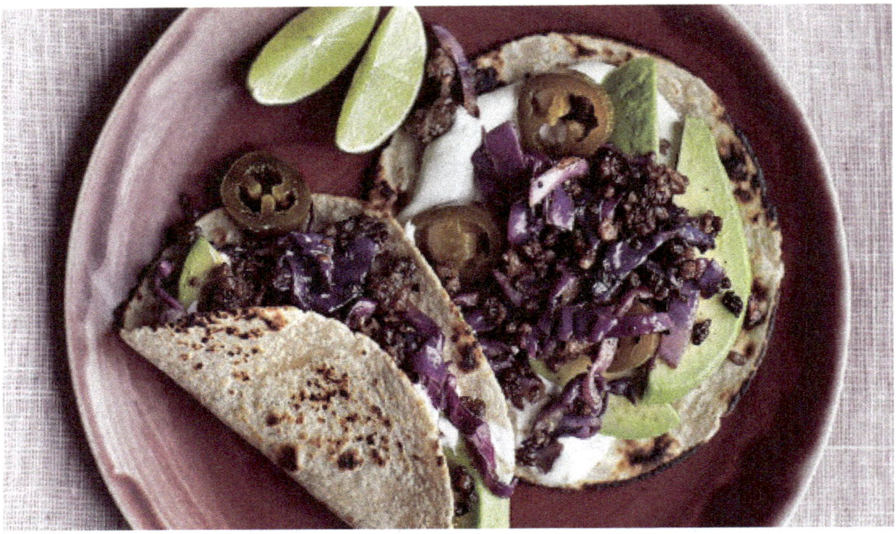

Preparation time: 10 Minutes

Cooking time: 15 Minutes

Servings: 4

Ingredients:

- Ground beef (1 lb.)
- Salsa - exPace Organic (.5 cup)
- Shredded cabbage (2 cups)
- Chili powder (2 tsp.)
- Shredded cheese (.75 cup)

Directions:

1. Brown the beef and drain the fat. Pour in the salsa, cabbage, and seasoning.
2. Cover and lower the heat. Simmer for 10 to 12 minutes using the medium heat temperature setting.
3. When the cabbage has softened, remove it from the heat and mix in the cheese.
4. Top it off using your favorite toppings, such as green onions or sour cream, and serve.

Nutrition:

- Calories: 325 Net Carbohydrates: 4g
- Protein Counts: 30g Total Fats: 21g

Creamy Pork Stew

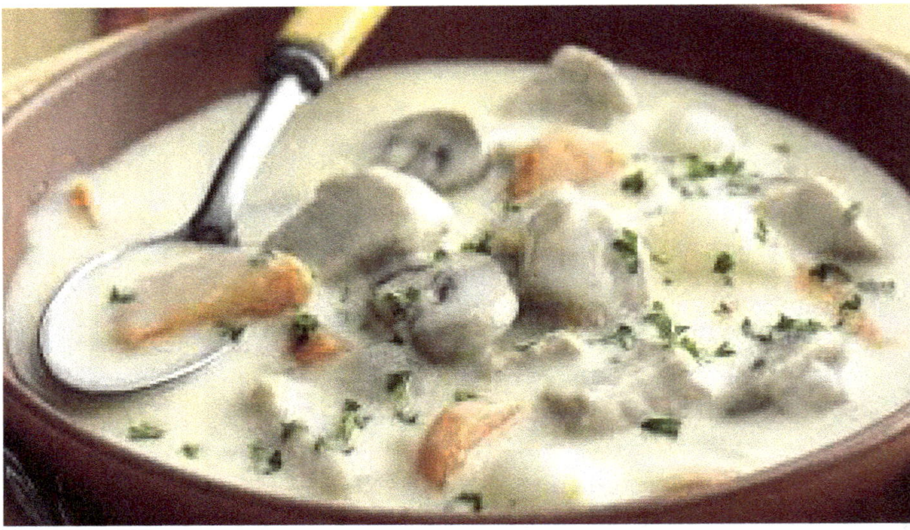

Preparation time: 15 Minutes

Cooking time: 1 Hour 35 minutes

Servings: 8

Ingredients:

- 3 Tbsp. unsalted butter
- 2½ Pounds boneless pork ribs
- 1 Yellow onion
- 4 Garlic cloves
- 1½ Cups chicken broth
- 2 Cans sugar-free diced tomatoes
- 2 Tsp. dried oregano
- 1 Tsp. ground cumin

- Salt
- 2 tbsp. lime juice
- ½ Cup sour cream

Directions:

1. Cook the pork, onions, and garlic within 4–5 minutes.
2. Add the broth, tomatoes, oregano, cumin, and salt, and mix. Simmer to low.
3. Combine in the sour cream plus lime juice and remove. Serve.

Nutrition:

- Calories: 304 Net Carbs: 4.7g
- Total Fat: 12.4g Protein: 39.5g

Salmon & Shrimp Stew

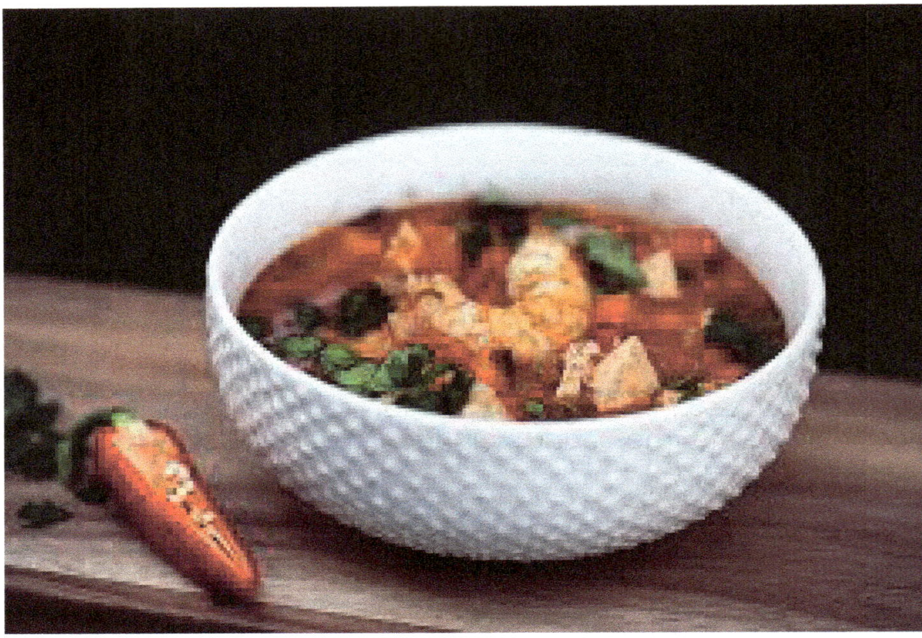

Preparation time: 20 Minutes

Cooking time: 25 Minutes

Servings: 6

Ingredients:

- 2 Tbsp coconut oil
- ½ Cup onion
- 2 Garlic cloves
- 1 Serrano pepper
- 1 Tsp. smoked paprika
- 24 Cups tomatoes
- 4 Cups chicken broth
- 1 Pound salmon fillets

- 1 Pound shrimp
- 2 Tbsp. lime juice
- Salt
- Ground black pepper
- 3 Tablespoons parsley

Directions:

1. Sauté the onion within 5–6 minutes. Add the garlic, Serrano pepper, and paprika. Add the tomatoes and broth, then boil. Simmer within 5 minutes. Add the salmon and simmer again, 3–4 minutes.
2. Put in the shrimp, then cook within 4–5 minutes. Mix in lemon juice, salt plus black pepper, and remove. Serve with parsley.

Nutrition:

- Calories: 247 Net Carbs: 3.9g
- Fiber: 1.2g Sugar: 2.1g Protein: 32.7g

Dessert Recipes

Raspberry Mousse

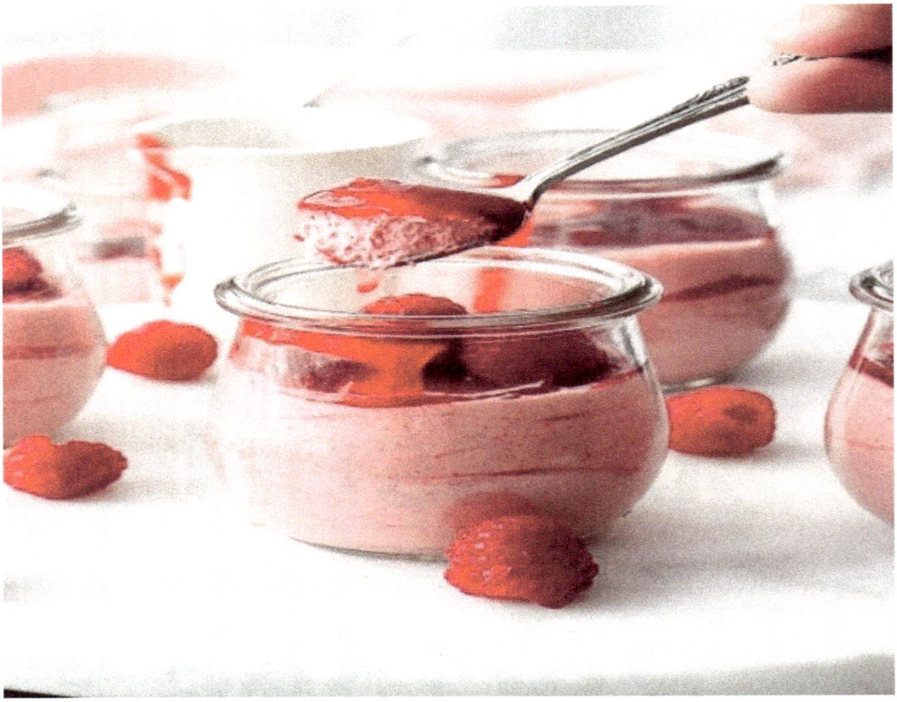

Preparation time: 10 Minutes

Cooking time: 4 Hours

Servings: 8

Ingredients:

- 3oz. Fresh raspberry
- 2 Cups heavy whipping cream
- 2oz. Pecans, chopped
- ¼ Tsp vanilla extract
- ½ Lemon, the zest

Directions:

1. Pour the whipping cream into the dish and blend until it becomes soft.
2. Put the lemon zest and vanilla into the dish and mix thoroughly.
3. Put the raspberries and nuts into the cream mix and stir well.
4. Cover the dish with plastic wrap and put it in the fridge for 3 hours.
5. Top with raspberries and serve.

Nutrition:

- Carbohydrates: 3g
- Fat: 26g
- Protein: 2g
- Calories: 255

Vanilla Crème Brûlée

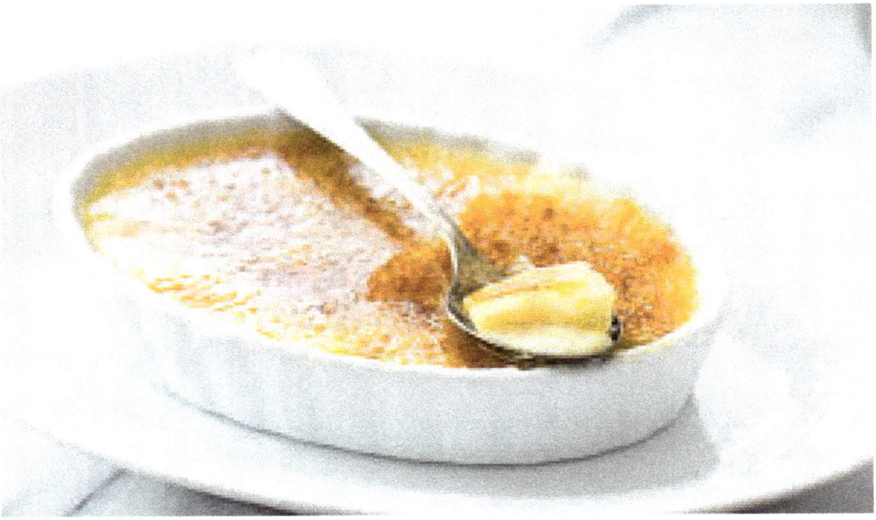

Preparation time: 20 Minutes

Cooking time: 1 Hour 20 minutes

Servings: 4

Ingredients:

- 2 Cups heavy cream
- 1 Vanilla bean, halved with seeds scraped out
- 4 Organic egg yolks
- 1/3 Teaspoon stevia powder
- 1 Teaspoon organic vanilla extract
- Pinch of salt
- 4 Tablespoon granulated erythritol

Directions:

1. Preheat your oven to 350°F.
2. In a pan, add heavy cream over medium heat and cook until heated.
3. Stir in the vanilla bean seeds and bring to a gentle boil.
4. Reduce the heat to very low and cook, covered for about 20 minutes.
5. Meanwhile, in a bowl, add the remaining ingredients (except erythritol) and beat until thick and pale mixture forms.
6. Remove the heavy cream from heat and through a fine-mesh strainer, strain into a heat-proof bowl.
7. Slowly add the cream to the egg yolk mixture beating continuously until well combined.
8. Divide the mixture into four ramekins evenly. Arrange the ramekins into a large baking dish. In the baking dish, add hot water, about half of the ramekins.
9. Bake for about 30–35 minutes.
10. Remove the pan from the oven and then let it cool slightly.
11. Refrigerate the ramekins for at least 4 hours.
12. Just before serving, sprinkle the ramekins with erythritol evenly.
13. Holding a kitchen torch about 4–5-inches from the top, caramelize the erythritol for about 2 minutes. Set aside for 5 minutes before serving.

Nutrition:

- Calories: 264 Fat: 26.7g
- Carbs: 2.4g Protein: 3.9g

Lemon Soufflé

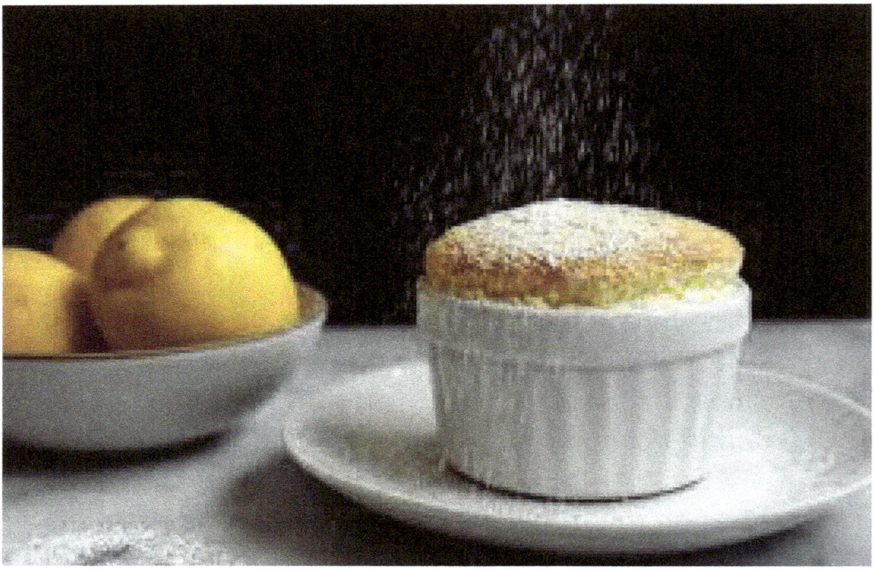

Preparation time: 15 Minutes

Cooking time: 35 Minutes

Servings: 4

Ingredients:

- 2 Large organic eggs (whites and yolks separated)
- ¼ Cups granulated erythritol, divided
- 1 Cup ricotta cheese
- 1 Tablespoon fresh lemon juice
- 2 Teaspoons lemon zest, grated
- 1 Teaspoon poppy seeds
- 1 Teaspoon organic vanilla extract

Directions:

1. Preheat your oven to 375ºF.
2. Grease 4 ramekins.
3. Add egg whites and beat in a clean glass bowl until it has a foam like texture.
4. Add two tablespoons of erythritol and beat the mixture until it is stiff.
5. In another bowl, add ricotta cheese, egg yolks, and the remaining erythritol until it is mixed thoroughly.
6. Put the lemon juice and lemon zest in the bowl and mix well.
7. Add the poppy seeds and vanilla extract and mix again.
8. Add the whipped egg whites into the ricotta mixture and gently stir.
9. Place the mixture into prepared ramekins evenly.
10. Bake for about 20 minutes.
11. Remove from the oven and serve immediately.

Nutrition:

- Calories: 130
- Fat: 7.7g
- Carbs: 4g
- Protein: 10.4g

Condiment Recipes

Cashew Cheese Sauce

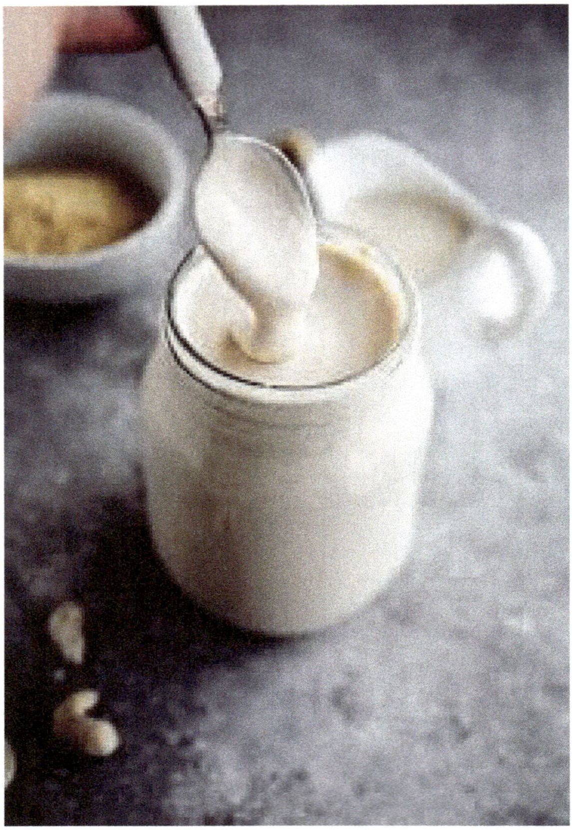

Preparation time: 5 Minutes

Cooking time: 0 Minutes

Servings: 8

Ingredients:

- 1 Tablespoon olive oil
- ½ Cup water
- ¾ Cup raw cashews
- 1 Tablespoon lemon juice

- ½ Teaspoon tamari sauce
- Salt

Directions:

1. As you begin a plant-based diet, you may be thinking you will miss your cheese. Luckily, this cashew cheese is an excellent replacement!
2. All you will have to do is take the rest of the components, place them into a blender, and combine until completely smoothed out.
3. Once you are done, place it in the fridge and enjoy!

Nutrition:

- Calories: 80
- Carbs: 11g
- Fat: 3g
- Protein: 2g

Balsamic Vinaigrette Dressing

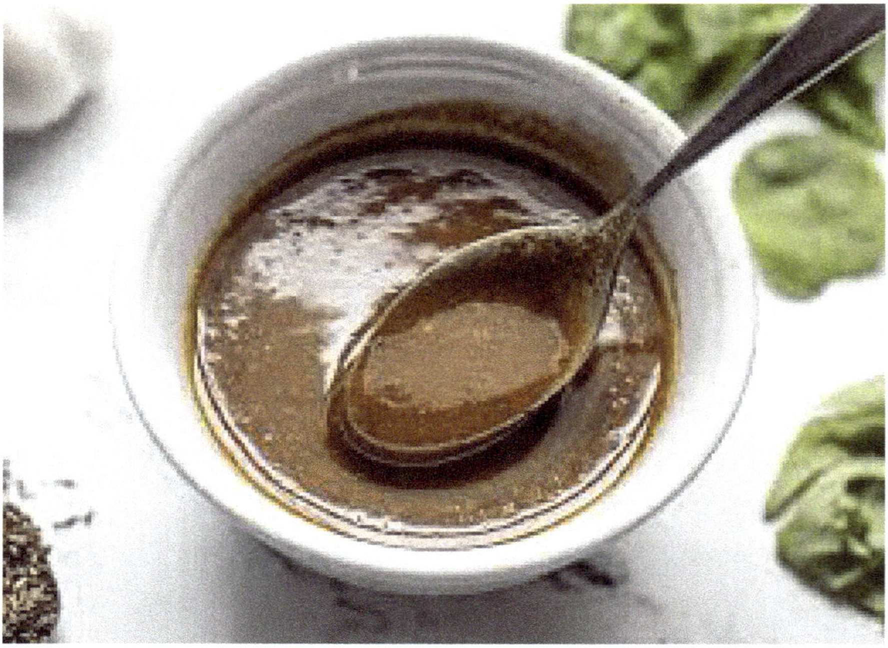

Preparation time: 5 Minutes

Cooking time: 0 Minute

Servings: 12

Ingredients:

- 1 Tablespoon garlic
- ¼ Cup olive oil
- ½ Teaspoon pepper
- ¼ Teaspoon cayenne pepper
- 1 Teaspoon salt

- 1 Tablespoon Dijon mustard
- ¼ Cup balsamic vinegar

Directions:

1. Looking for a light salad dressing? Take all the ingredients, place them in a mixer, and mix until smoothed out.
2. Store up in the fridge and enjoy over any salad!

Nutrition:

- Calories: 50
- Carbs: 3g
- Fat: 4g
- Protein: 0g

Salad Recipes

Cauliflower Salad

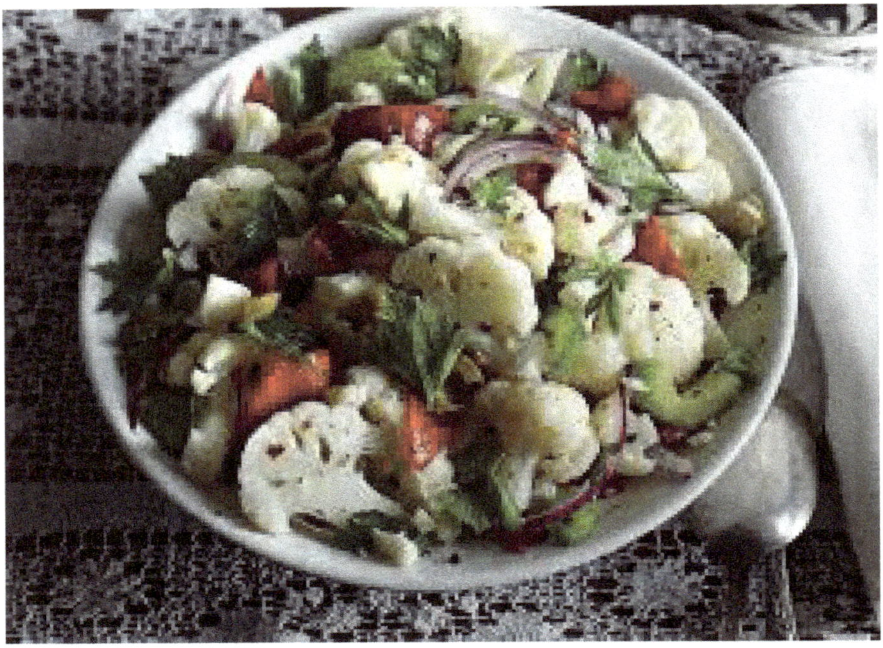

Preparation time: 10 Minutes

Cooking time: 0 Minutes

Servings: 4

Ingredients:

- 2 Tablespoons olive oil
- 1 Cup black olives, pitted and halved
- 6 Cups cauliflower florets, grated and blanched
- Salt and ground black pepper, to taste
- ¼ Cup onion, chopped
- 1 Teaspoon fresh mint leaves, chopped
- 1 Tablespoon fresh parsley, chopped
- Juice of ½ lemon

Directions:

1. In a salad bowl, mix the cauliflower with the olives and the other ingredients, toss and serve.

Nutrition:

- Calories per serving: 860
- Carbohydrates: 6g
- Protein: 10.5g
- Fat: 6g
- Sugar: 1g
- Sodium: 604mg
- Fiber: 1g

Wedge Salad

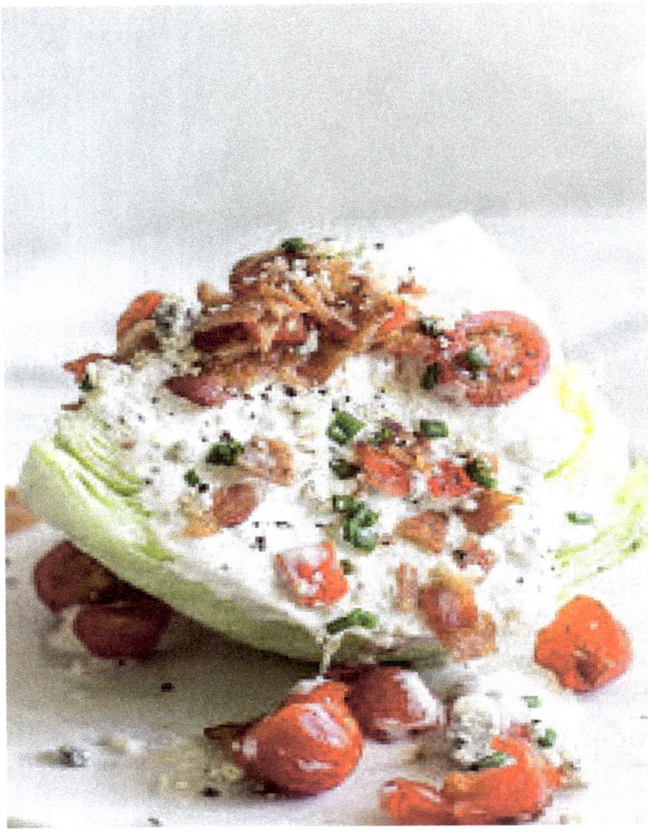

Preparation time: 10 Minutes

Cooking time: 10 Minutes

Servings: 2

Ingredients:

- 4 Bacon slices
- ½ Head iceberg lettuce halved
- Two tablespoons blue cheese salad dressing (I use Trader Joe's Chunky Blue Cheese Dressing)

- ¼ Cup blue cheese crumbles
- ½ Cup halved grape tomatoes

Directions:

1. In a large skillet over medium-high heat, cook the bacon on both sides until crispy, about 8 minutes. Transfer the bacon to a paper towel-lined plate to drain and cool for 5 minutes. Transfer to a cutting board and chop the bacon.
2. Place the lettuce wedges on two plates. Top each with half of the blue cheese dressing, the blue cheese crumbles, the halved grape tomatoes, and the chopped bacon, and serve.
3. If you have a grill, you can drizzle each of your iceberg lettuce wedges with one tablespoon of olive oil, season with pink Himalayan salt and pepper, and grill each side for about 1 minute to add some smoky flavor. Then dress the lettuce wedges as instructed.

Nutrition:

- Calories: 278
- Total Fat: 20g
- Carbs: 9g
- Net Carbs: 7g
- Fiber: 3g
- Protein: 15g

Alternative Bread Recipe

Oatmeal Zucchini Bread

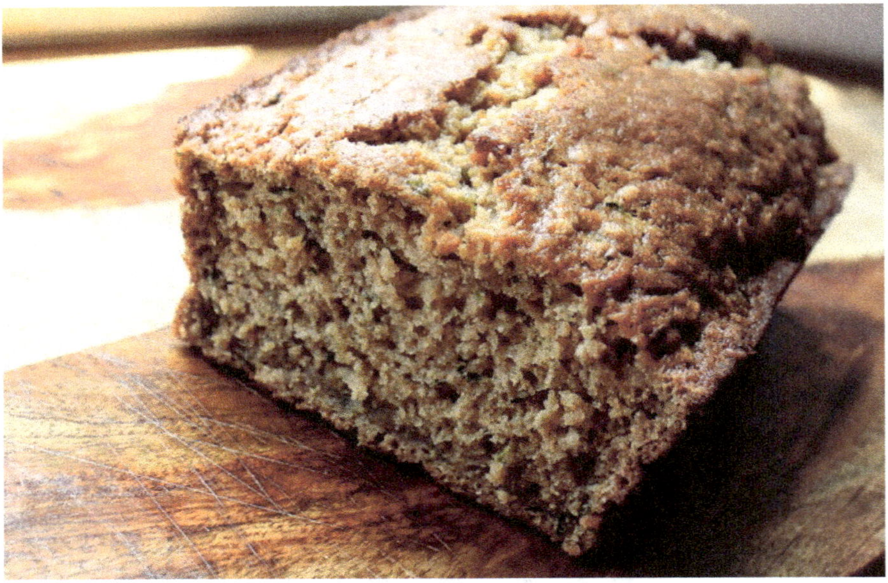

Preparation time: 10 Minutes

Cooking time: 20-30 Minutes

Servings: 1 loaf

Ingredients:

- ⅓ Cup milk, at 80°F to 90°F
- ½ Cup finely shredded zucchini
- ¼ Teaspoon freshly squeezed lemon juice, at room temperature
- 2 Teaspoons olive oil
- 2 Teaspoons sugar
- ⅔ Teaspoon salt
- ½ Cup quick oats
- ½ Cup whole-wheat flour

- 1 Cup white bread flour
- 1½ Teaspoons bread machine or instant yeast

Directions:

1. Place the ingredients in your bread machine as recommended by the manufacturer.
2. Program the machine for Basic/White bread, select light or medium crust, and press Start.
3. When the loaf is done, remove the bucket from the machine.
4. Let the loaf cool for 5 minutes.
5. Gently shake the bucket to remove the loaf and turn it out onto a rack to cool.

Nutrition:

- Calories: 127
- Total Fat: 2g
- Saturated Fat: 0g
- Carbohydrates: 23g
- Fiber: 1g
- Sodium: 200mg
- Protein: 4g

Appetizers and Snacks

Brussels Sprouts and Bacon

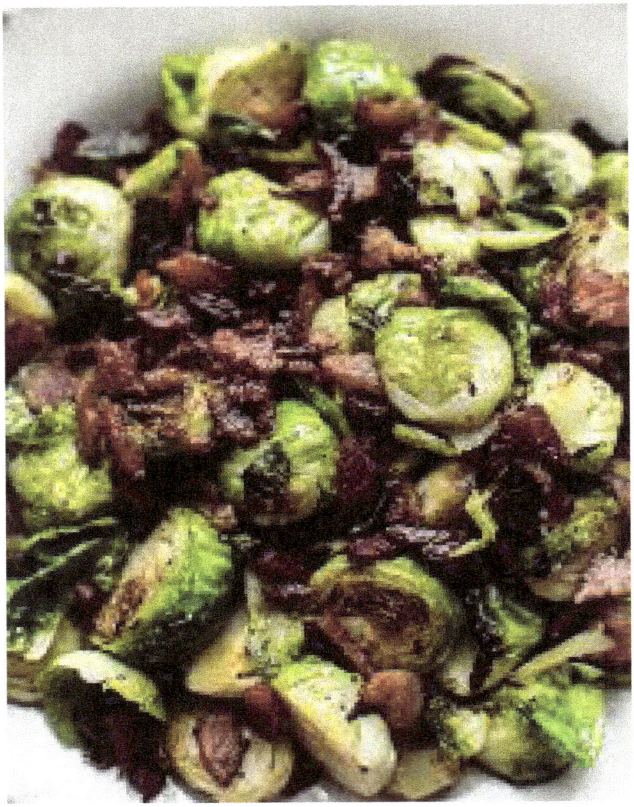

Preparation time: 10 Minutes

Cooking time: 30 Minutes

Servings: 4

Ingredients:

- 8 Bacon strips, chopped
- 1 Pound Brussels sprouts, trimmed and halved
- Salt and ground black pepper, to taste
- A pinch of cumin

- A pinch of red pepper, crushed
- 2 Tablespoons extra virgin olive oil

Directions:

1. In a bowl, mix the Brussels sprouts with salt, pepper, cumin, red pepper, and oil, and toss to coat.
2. Spread the Brussels sprouts on a lined baking sheet, place in an oven at 375ºF, and bake for 30 minutes.
3. Heat a pan over medium heat, add the bacon pieces, and cook them until they become crispy.
4. Divide the baked Brussels sprouts on plates, top with bacon, and serve.

Nutrition:

- Calories: 256
- Fat: 20g
- Fiber: 6g
- Carbohydrates: 5g
- Protein: 15g

Creamy Spinach

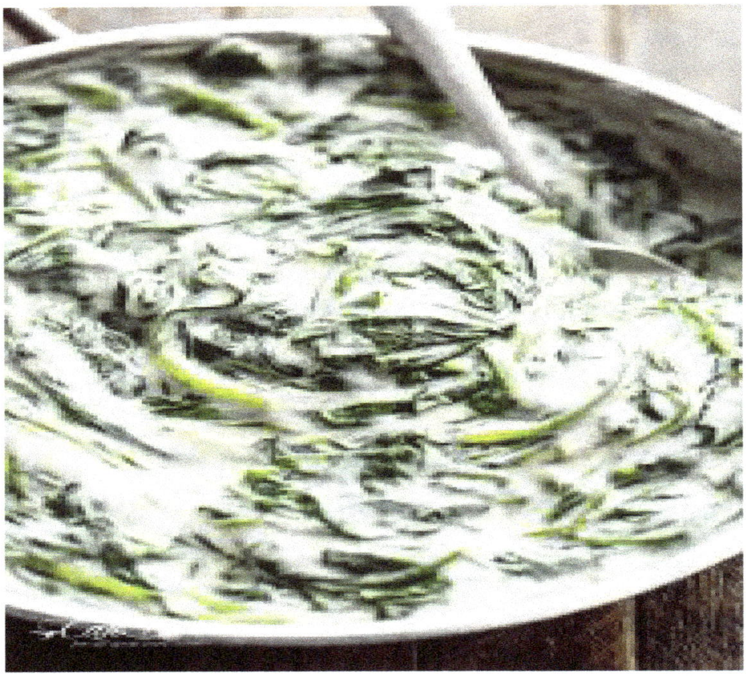

Preparation time: 10 Minutes

Cooking time: 15 Minutes

Servings: 2

Ingredients:

- 2 Garlic cloves, peeled and minced
- 8 Ounces of spinach leaves
- A drizzle of olive oil
- Salt and ground black pepper, to taste
- 4 Tablespoons sour cream

- 1 Tablespoon butter
- 2 Tablespoons Parmesan cheese, grated

Directions:

1. Heat a pan with the oil over medium heat, add the spinach, stir and cook until it softens.
2. Add the salt, pepper, butter, Parmesan cheese, and butter, stir, and cook for 4 minutes.
3. Add the sour cream, stir, and cook for 5 minutes.
4. Divide between plates and serve.

Nutrition:

- Calories: 233
- Fat: 10g
- Fiber: 4g
- Carbohydrates: 4g
- Protein: 2g

Avocado Fries

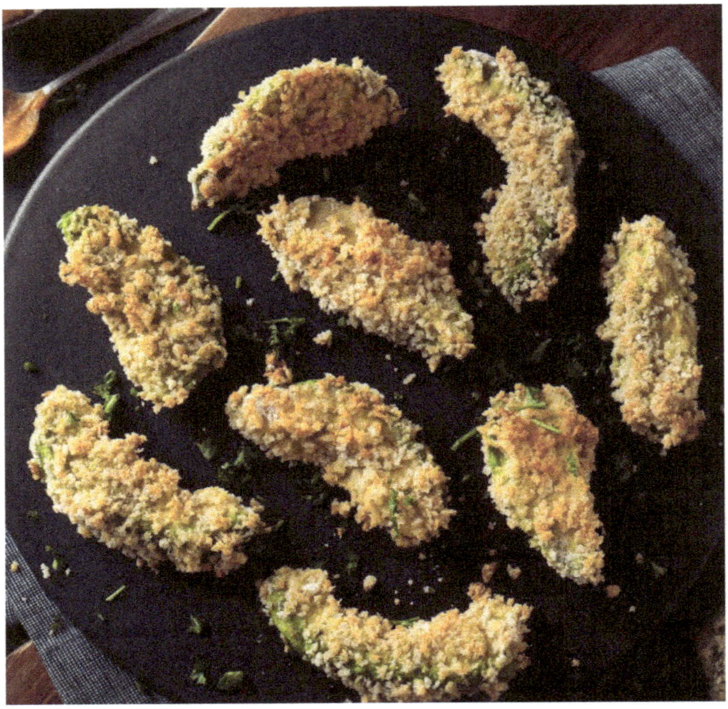

Preparation time: 10 Minutes

Cooking time: 5 Minutes

Servings: 3

Ingredients:

- 3 Avocados, pitted, peeled, halved, and sliced
- 1½ Cups sunflower oil
- 1½ Cups almond meal
- A pinch of cayenne pepper

- Salt and ground black pepper, to taste

Directions:

1. In a bowl, mix the almond meal with salt, pepper, and cayenne, and stir. In a second bowl, whisk eggs with a pinch of salt and pepper.
2. Dredge the avocado pieces in the whisked eggs and then in almond meal mixture. Heat a pan with the oil over medium-high heat, add the avocado fries, and cook them until they are golden.
3. Transfer to paper towels, drain grease and divide between plates to serve.

Nutrition:

- Calories: 200
- Fat: 43g
- Fiber: 4g
- Carbs: 7g
- Protein: 17g

About the author

Dana Roberts is an author, nutritionist and mom of three beautiful princesses.
At the age of 38 she discovered that she had breast disease and this brought her a big hormonal imbalance.
At the age of 43 she noticed a gradual weight gain that prompted her to try different diets.
So many of these had little or no effect on her. After a few years, her body underwent drastic changes.
She gained a lot of weight, her breasts collapsed and a lot of stretch marks appeared. Not wanting to risk serious health problems, she discovered the ketogenic diet and decided to try it.
She began to notice that some foods gave her more energy and others weighed her down. Food addiction also influenced her diet because when she didn't bring awareness to her emotions, she reacted by eating.
She spent years fighting this addiction and finally found a way to overcome it and rediscover her former beauty, creating recipes that could fill both her stomach and her soul.
The book "Keto Diet Cookbook for women after 50" offers to all women the possibility to lose weight with a program based not only on diet, but also on the addiction that sometimes food creates.

CPSIA information can be obtained
at www.ICGtesting.com
Printed in the USA
BVHW012356020321
601387BV00026B/519

9 781914 085253